ScrubTales™ Surgical Technologist

A Real-World Career Guide That Tells the Truth About the Operating Room and Surgical Teamwork

ScrubTales™ Series 1 — Core Clinical Careers

Mason Preddy

MASON MAISON
PUBLISHING™
REWRITING THE NARRATIVE
MASONMAISON.PUB

MASON MAISON
PUBLISHING™
REWRITING THE NARRATIVE
MASONMAISON.PUB

This book is published by Mason Maison™ Publishing.

The information contained in this book is provided for educational and informational purposes only. While every effort has been made to ensure accuracy at the time of publication, healthcare careers, credentialing requirements, compensation ranges, regulatory standards, and professional expectations may change over time and vary by location, employer, and governing body. Readers are encouraged to verify all information with appropriate educational institutions, certification organizations, licensing boards, professional associations, and employers before making career or educational decisions.

This book does not provide medical, legal, financial, or career-placement advice, nor does it guarantee employment, compensation outcomes, licensure eligibility, admission to training programs, or career advancement. Individual experiences, hiring outcomes, workplace environments, and financial results may vary widely based on personal qualifications, geographic region, institutional policies, and market conditions.

Any references to organizations, employers, products, technologies, or clinical environments are provided for illustrative or educational purposes only and do not constitute endorsement.

By using this book, the reader acknowledges responsibility for their own professional, educational, and career decisions.

“Most people never see the hands that lay out the tools, guard the sterile space, and steady the quiet seconds between fear and repair. But every life that leaves the operating room safer than it entered carries their fingerprints too.”

Chapter 1
Welcome

If you're holding this book, there's a good chance you're the kind of person who notices details other people miss. You straighten crooked lines. You like when things click into place. You care about getting it right. Somewhere along the way, someone may have told you, "You'd be great in the OR," or you've watched a surgery clip and thought, "I want to be in that room." This book is for you.

It's for the student who's tired of vague career advice and wants to know what it *actually* feels like to stand at the surgical field, hands ready, eyes on the sterile tray. It's for the high school senior who keeps Googling healthcare careers and getting the same generic blurbs over and over. It's for the career changer who's done being bored at a desk and is wondering what it would be like to walk into a hospital instead of a cubicle. It's for the allied health or pre-nursing student who suspects, deep down, that the operating room might be where they really come alive.

It's also for the people who care about you: the parent trying to understand what their kid wants to do with their life, the teacher advising students on healthcare pathways, the counselor, advisor, or mentor who wants something more concrete than a one-page job description. If you're trying to figure out whether the Surgical Technologist role is a genuine, sustainable match for you—or for someone you're helping—this book is your alignment check.

This is not a fantasy version of the job. Surgical technology is not just matching instruments to a surgeon's hand in perfectly lit, slow-motion scenes. It's sweat under your sterile gown, learning to read the room without a word, being ready for the moment a routine case suddenly isn't routine anymore. It's the quiet satisfaction of having the exact clamp ready before the surgeon even asks. It's the frustration of being overlooked or misunderstood by people who don't really know what you do. It's the physical strain, the early mornings, the long cases, and the emotional weight of seeing people on some of the hardest days of their lives.

That's why this book is honest. You deserve more than a brochure and a pep talk. You deserve a clear picture of the pace, the pressure, the politics, and the payoff. We talk about the hard parts: standing for hours, the hierarchy in the OR, the reality of nights, weekends, holidays, and call. We talk about when it feels like magic and when it absolutely does not. We talk about the difference between what schools, recruiters, and glossy websites highlight—and what your body and mind will actually live through in this role.

Honest doesn't mean harsh. It means respectful. It means treating you like an adult who can hold complexity: that you can love the work *and* admit it's exhausting, that you can be proud of your skills *and* know this role isn't for everyone. The goal of this book is not to push you into becoming a Surgical Technologist at all costs. The goal is to align you—your wiring, your values, your energy—with work that fits. If surgical technology is that fit, this book will help you see it clearly. If it's not, this book will help you figure that out before you enroll, sign, or commit.

You can use this book two ways: quick skim or deep dive. Both are valid; it depends on where you are and how much time and headspace you have right now.

If you're in skim mode, think of this book as a fast, honest radar scan. Start with the sections that give you the "big picture first" view—the parts that answer: Who does well in this role? What does a typical day feel like? What does it cost you, and what does it give you back? As you skim, pay attention to your body. Do you feel yourself leaning in, curious, wanting more? Or do you feel a quiet, uncomfortable "nope" that you're tempted to ignore because it sounds impressive to say you work in surgery? That reaction matters.

Skimming is ideal if you're comparing multiple careers and trying to narrow your list. Use the big narrative moments and the alignment-style sections as a filter: could you see yourself in this story, or do you feel like you're watching someone else's life from far away? You don't have to highlight every other sentence. You're just looking for a gut-level sense of "close" or "not quite."

If you're ready for a deeper dive, this book becomes more like a guided reflection. Read it slowly, cover to cover if you can. Pause after the more intense or detailed sections and ask yourself real questions: Do I want this level of responsibility? How do I handle pressure now, in school or work? What kind of teamwork brings out the best in me—and what kind drains me? Where do I see myself in five years, not just in title, but in how my life feels?

As you read deeply, imagine a real shift, not a movie montage. Picture the alarm going off at 04:45 for a long day of cases. Picture the first time you scrub in on a procedure that runs three hours longer than expected. Picture how it might feel to leave a shift knowing you did your job well—and how it might feel to drive home after a tough day, replaying a moment that didn't go the way you wanted. Let the narrative help you practice those feelings before you're in the middle of them.

You can also use this book as a conversation starter. Bring specific pages to a teacher, advisor, or mentor and say, "This part really sounded like me," or "This section describes a type of stress I'm not sure I could handle." Use it with a parent who's worried you're choosing something "too intense," or with a partner who wants to understand why this work matters to you. Real career decisions are rarely made alone; this book is designed to give everyone a clearer, shared picture.

And finally, you can use this book as a mirror over time. Come back to it when your circumstances change: when you finish a clinical rotation, after your first job interview, after a tough semester, or when you're considering a shift in direction. What once felt thrilling might start to feel heavy; what once felt intimidating might begin to feel like a healthy challenge. Alignment isn't a one-time event. It's something you check, recheck, and adjust as you grow.

You are not "too picky" for wanting a career that fits. You are not unrealistic for wanting to know the truth about what you're walking into. This book exists because your time, your energy, and your future patients deserve a good match—not just a good story. If surgical technology ends up being your lane, you'll know it because the picture in these pages will feel familiar long before you ever step into your first OR. If it's not your lane, you'll still walk away with more clarity, more language for what *does* fit you, and more confidence in the choices you make next.

However you choose to use this book—quick skim, slow study, or something in between—treat it as a tool, not a test. You're not trying to pass. You're trying to discover whether this path lines up with who you are and who you're becoming. That's the real work here. And you're already doing it.

Chapter 2

A Note to the Reader

You'll notice certain terms in this book marked with **(gl)** — these are glossary terms. Healthcare has a language of its own, and I've included a glossary at the end of this book so you can look up any unfamiliar phrases along the way.

As a special bonus, that glossary also highlights additional key terms every aspiring Surgical Technologist should know — especially if you plan to build a long-term career in the operating room. It's a great place to start building fluency in the language of sterile technique, instrumentation, and real-world teamwork in surgery.

As always, I wish you great success in whatever career aligns with you.

Chapter 3

What This Career Really Is

The lights above you hum softly as the clock creeps toward 06:55. The air in the operating room (gl) feels cool and almost too bright, every surface wiped, every edge shining. On your back table (gl), the instruments you opened and arranged before sunrise rest in neat rows: clamps, scissors, needle holders, forceps. You've checked them twice already. The sterile (gl) drapes are folded just so, stacked in the order you'll need them. Your gown and gloves are ready for you to scrub in (gl), waiting for that first case of the day.

The patient rolls in, eyes a little wide, heart rate flickering across the monitor. Anesthesia (gl) starts their calm ritual, placing monitor leads, checking blood pressure, confirming medications. The surgeon steps into the room, glances at the schedule, then at your setup. You can tell from the way their shoulders drop a fraction: they see that every instrument is exactly where it should be. You've built a tiny, precise world on that Mayo stand (gl), and they're about to trust you with it.

After you scrub in, your hands rise in front of you, fingers pointed to the ceiling like you've practiced a hundred times. Someone helps you into your gown and pulls your gloves on without breaking the sterile field (gl). When the patient is draped, the room shifts. Small talk stops. The surgeon calls for the first instrument. Without looking down, you place it into their waiting hand in one smooth motion. You already know the next three things they'll probably ask for.

The first incision (gl) is small, almost delicate, but the moment it's made, everything becomes more serious. Suction whirs quietly. A retractor (gl) slides into place to open up the view. The anesthetist adjusts medications. Electrocautery (gl) pops and sizzles softly in the background. You are close enough to see the smallest details, but your job is not to watch in awe. Your job is to think ahead, anticipate, and protect the sterile space that makes the entire surgery possible.

An hour later, the room looks different: used sponges pile up in their designated spot, instruments rest in different positions, the wound begins to close. You're counting out loud with the circulating nurse (gl), making sure every sponge, needle, and instrument that went in has been accounted for. When the final suture (gl) is tied and the dressing is placed, there is a quiet moment of satisfaction that no one outside this room will ever see. The surgeon gets the credit; the patient gets the result. You get the knowledge that the case ran smoothly because you were there, steady and prepared, from wheels in to wheels out.

That is the heart of surgical technology. A Surgical Technologist (gl), sometimes called a "scrub tech" or "surgical tech," is the person who prepares the operating room before a case, sets up the instruments and supplies, maintains the sterile field, and passes instruments during surgery. You are the bridge between the carefully packed trays from sterile processing (gl) and the surgeon's hands. You are the one who helps make sure nothing is missing, nothing is contaminated, and nothing is left behind.

In this role, you become an expert in the flow of surgery. You learn the steps of common procedures so well that you can anticipate the next move without anyone saying a word. You understand how to position equipment, how to open and organize trays, how to keep your field clean, and how to respond when something unexpected happens. You are not "just handing instruments." You are actively managing risk, efficiency, and safety in every case.

You are also part of the larger perioperative (gl) team, working alongside surgeons, anesthesiologists (gl), nurse anesthetists (gl), circulating nurses, and other staff. While the surgeon may lead the procedure, the quality of the entire experience for the patient depends on how well the whole team works together. A strong Surgical Technologist is a quiet force for order in a high-stakes environment. You are the person who notices the missing item, the small break in technique, or the subtle shift in the room that says, "Something's not right."

Chapter 4

Pros and Cons of becoming a Surgical Technologist

Pros

- You are close to the action in every case. If you want to be right there at the surgical field, not watching from a window or a video screen, this role gives you a front-row position. You see anatomy in real time, watch problems get fixed, and participate in moments most people only see on television. For many Surgical Technologists, that sense of proximity to real, life-changing work never stops feeling meaningful.

- You build a very specific, valuable skill set. Not many people know how to maintain strict sterile technique (gl), anticipate a surgeon's needs, or manage complex instrument setups under pressure. Those are not generic skills; they are specialized and highly respected inside the OR (gl) world. As you gain experience, you become the person people trust when they want a smooth, efficient case.

- You can enter the field relatively quickly. Compared to some healthcare careers that require many years of school, Surgical

Technologist programs are often shorter, allowing you to get into the workforce faster. That means you can start earning, learning, and deciding how much you like the OR (gl) environment sooner. If you later choose to advance to other roles, your hands-on experience will be a strong foundation.

- Your work has a direct impact on patient safety. Accurate counts, good sterile practice, and well-organized setups are not “extras”; they are safety barriers that protect real people. When you prevent a contamination, catch a missing instrument, or speak up about an error, you are directly preventing harm. That connection to safety can be deeply satisfying for people who care about doing things the right way.

- You are part of a tight-knit team. OR (gl) teams tend to be smaller and more familiar than some other hospital units. Over time, you get to know the surgeons, nurses, and anesthesia providers you work with on a daily basis. When the team is healthy, that closeness can create a strong sense of belonging, shared humor, and pride in how well you work together.

- There is variety in procedures and specialties. You might assist with orthopedic cases one day, general surgery the next, and then move into specialties like neurosurgery (gl), cardiovascular surgery (gl), or plastics as your career evolves. Each specialty has its own rhythm, instruments, and challenges. This variety helps prevent boredom and allows you to explore what kind of cases you enjoy most.

- You can grow into roles beyond the field. Experienced Surgical Technologists can move into positions like preceptor (gl), lead tech, OR (gl) coordinator, or roles in sterile processing (gl) and vendor (gl) services. Some go on to nursing, physician assistant, or other advanced clinical careers, bringing their OR insight with them. The skills you build here can open doors you may not see yet.

Cons

- You spend long hours on your feet. Many surgeries last far longer than the schedule suggests, and you may be standing in one place for most of that time. Your back, legs, and feet will feel it, especially if you are not careful about shoes, posture, and self-care. If you dislike physical strain or can't tolerate standing for extended periods, this role may wear you down.

- The schedule can be demanding and unpredictable. ORs run early, and some run late. You may be expected to take call (gl), come in for emergency cases at night, or stay when a procedure runs long. Holidays, weekends, and off-hours work are common. If you highly value a predictable 9-to-5 schedule, this career can clash with how you want your life to feel.

- The OR culture can be intense. Surgical environments are known for strong personalities, high expectations, and a focus on speed and precision. You may encounter raised voices, impatience, or perfectionism that feels personal even when it's not. If you are very sensitive to criticism or conflict, the emotional side of this work may be exhausting.

- You may feel invisible to the outside world. Patients rarely remember your name, and many people outside healthcare do not understand what you do. The surgeon often receives the public thanks and recognition, even when your work was critical to the outcome. If you need visible credit or frequent external validation, this behind-the-scenes role might feel discouraging.

• You must tolerate blood, body fluids, and difficult cases. You will see real bodies, real injuries, and real complications. Some cases involve trauma, amputations, or cancer. Even "routine" surgeries can have unexpected outcomes. If you are easily overwhelmed by graphic scenes or medical distress, this reality can be hard to carry over time.

• The margin for error is small. A missed count, a contaminated instrument, or a detail that slips by can have serious consequences. Most days go smoothly, but when something goes wrong, it feels heavy. If you struggle with anxiety or have a hard time letting go of mistakes, you may find the mental load of this role particularly challenging.

• Turnover (gl) and pressure for speed can be relentless. Hospitals push for quick room turnovers and high efficiency. You may feel rushed to prepare for the next case while still mentally processing the last one. When volume is high, it can feel like there is never quite enough time to breathe, reset, or debrief.

This career is for you if...

• You feel energized by fast-paced, high-stakes environments where your focus and preparation matter.

• You like working with your hands and enjoy arranging, organizing, and fine-tuning physical tools and setups.

- You are good at paying attention to details and can notice small changes or missing items quickly.

- You can handle direct feedback and occasional stress without taking everything personally.

- You are comfortable supporting others' leadership while owning your part of the process with pride.

- You care deeply about safety and are willing to speak up when something seems off, even if it's awkward.

- You like routines but don't mind when a day takes a sharp turn and you have to adapt.

- You want a career where you can see the impact of your work, even if most people outside the room never know your name.

This career will frustrate you if...

- You strongly dislike being on your feet for long stretches or doing physically demanding work.

- You need a calm, quiet environment most of the time to feel okay.

- You want a predictable schedule with very few early mornings, late nights, weekends, or holidays.

- You prefer work where mistakes are low-stakes and you can take your time without pressure.

- You need frequent public recognition, praise, or visible titles to feel valued.

- You become easily discouraged by criticism, especially when it's delivered quickly or bluntly.

- You do not want to be around blood, open tissue, or the realities of surgery on a regular basis.
- You prefer to lead from the front rather than support from the side and may resent not being “the main” person in the room.

Chapter 5
What I Wish I Had Known

What I Wish I Had Known

Before you ever put on your first pair of hospital-issue scrubs (gl), it is easy to imagine this career as a straight line: go to school, get certified, get hired, scrub (gl) into surgery, feel proud forever. The truth is more complicated and more human. There are parts of this work that are more beautiful than you expect, and parts that are heavier, stranger, or more exhausting than anyone probably told you. If you end up loving it, it won't be because it was easy. It will be because you walked in with your eyes open and learned how to stay yourself in the middle of it all.

Here are some of the things many Surgical Technologists (gl) wish they had known at the beginning—things that could help you prepare your head and your heart, not just your hands.

I wish I had known that feeling clueless at first is normal, not proof I picked the wrong career.

In school, you can memorize every instrument name and still feel completely lost the first time you're in a real operating room (gl). The surgeon is speaking quickly, the anesthesiologist (gl) is giving updates, the circulating nurse (gl) is moving in and out of the room, and you're standing there thinking, "I know that clamp exists... I just cannot find it in this mountain of metal."

What nobody says clearly enough is that this disorientation is part of the process, not a personal failure. Every hospital has different preference cards (gl), different brands of instruments, different ways of setting up a back table. You are learning a new language and a new kitchen at the same time.

If you expect to feel competent right away, you will be discouraged. If you expect to feel overwhelmed and treat that as a temporary phase, you will be patient with yourself. The goal in the beginning is not perfection; it is progress: one instrument you recognize faster, one setup that feels smoother, one case where you anticipate a step instead of reacting to it.

I wish I had known how much of this job is about people, not just procedures.

From the outside, it looks like your whole world will be instruments and sterile (gl) technique. And those things matter deeply. But the longer you work, the more you realize: you are in the relationship business as much as the surgical business.

You will work with surgeons who are calm and kind, and surgeons who are brilliant but sharp. You will work with nurses who feel like family, and others who test your patience. You will see anesthesiology providers who quietly save the day, and circulating nurses who protect the room's energy like it's their job—because it is.

You don't have to be a social butterfly to thrive, but you do need basic emotional skills: how to stay respectful when someone is short with you; how to apologize when you make a mistake; how to give a clear, calm report when something is wrong. You are part of a small team in a high-stakes box. The way you speak and listen matters as much as the way you pass a scalpel (gl).

Small story – "The surgeon who wasn't actually mean."

Early on, many techs meet "that" surgeon—the one everybody warns them about. You pass an instrument a beat too late, and they snap, "I need you with me, not behind." It stings. On break, you hear staff trade stories about their temper, and it is tempting to decide, "They hate me." Later, you learn that this same surgeon quietly buys coffee for night shift, or goes down to the ICU (intensive care unit) (gl) on their day off to check on a patient. You start to understand that people can be intense in the room and still care deeply. Learning to see the human behind the tone is part of growing up in this environment.

I wish I had known how physically demanding it really is.

You know, in theory, that you'll be on your feet. It still surprises many people how much your body is part of the job. You will stand in one position for long cases. You will hold retractors (gl) with your arms locked while your shoulders burn. You will push heavy beds, move case carts, and bend over to reach sterile supplies on low shelves.

Comfortable shoes help. Stretching helps. Hydrating helps. But the deeper truth is that you are signing up for physical work. If you take care of your body outside the hospital—sleep, food, movement—you will last longer inside it.

What nobody explains well enough is how closely your physical state and your focus are tied. It's hard to anticipate steps and notice contamination risks when your back feels like it's on fire and you haven't eaten in eight hours. Learning to manage your energy is not selfish; it is patient safety.

I wish I had known that some days the hardest part would be after the case, not during it.

In the moment, you are busy: counting sponges, passing clamps, watching the field. You do not have much room to feel anything beyond "What's next?" and "Is this safe?" The emotions often arrive later—walking out of the room, alone in the locker room, or lying in bed at night.

You will have cases where everything goes right and the patient still doesn't make it. You will have pediatric cases that stick with you longer than you expect. You will see trauma (gl) patients whose stories you cannot unsee. On those days, you may find yourself replaying the sequence again and again, wondering if you could have done something different, even when everyone tells you the outcome was unavoidable.

No one can completely prepare you for this, but knowing it is coming helps. You might need a ritual—taking a walk after work, journaling, talking to one trusted person who understands confidentiality (gl) and boundaries. You might need to give yourself permission to feel sad or shaken without labeling yourself as "too sensitive for this work." Being affected means your empathy is intact. The key is learning how to process it instead of letting it pile up.

Small story – "The first time the patient didn't wake up."

Many techs remember the first time a case ends and the patient does not go to recovery, because they did not survive the operation. The room gets very quiet. People move with a different kind of heaviness. You help clean, send instruments to be reprocessed (gl), and then the next case appears on the board as if nothing massive just happened. You might go home that night feeling like the world outside is out of sync—people are at the grocery store, kids are laughing in the parking lot, and you are carrying the image of a still body in a silent OR. Knowing that this disconnect is normal—and that it gets easier to carry with support—can keep you from feeling like you're "broken" for struggling with it.

I wish I had known how much small habits would shape my reputation.

It's easy to picture your reputation riding on big moments: the way you handle an emergency, how you respond when something goes wrong. In reality, most people form their opinion of you based on small, repeated behaviors.

Do you show up on time, ready to start your setup instead of wandering in at the last minute? Do you check your preference card before you scrub, or do you rely on everyone else to fix gaps? Do you help with turnover without being asked, or vanish the second your case is over? Do you talk about coworkers respectfully, or join in every bit of gossip?

Surgeons and nurses notice who keeps their word. Sterile processing staff notice who returns instruments in good condition. Charge nurses notice who can be trusted with harder rooms. Over time, these tiny choices add up to labels like "solid," "flaky," "sharp," or "lazy." You cannot control everything people say, but you have more power than you think over the patterns they see.

I wish I had known that advocacy is part of the job, even if you are not the one with the title.

You might think, "I'm just the tech; I don't make decisions." That mindset can get patients hurt. Part of your role is to speak up when something feels unsafe or off—even if you are the least experienced person in the room.

That might mean saying, "We did not get a closing count yet," even if everyone seems eager to move on. It might mean pointing out a contaminated (gl) glove or a sleeve that brushed the unsterile part of the bed. It might mean quietly asking, "Can we pause and re-check the site?" if something about the prep or the consent does not match what you heard.

You will not do this perfectly. There will be days you realize afterward that you noticed something and stayed silent. Those memories can burn. They can also become strong teachers. The sooner you accept that your eyes and voice matter, the sooner you become the kind of tech other people trust to help guard the line between "fine" and "we should have caught that."

I wish I had known that imposter syndrome doesn't magically go away—it just changes shape.

At the beginning, your doubts sound like, "I don't belong here. I'm going to mess up everything." Later, they become, "Why did they put me in this difficult room? I'm not ready," or, "Everyone else is handling this better than I am."

You might think that once you can set up a room in your sleep or recognize every instrument at a glance, you'll finally feel completely confident. The reality is that you just move the goalposts. As you get better, you are trusted with more complex cases, tougher surgeons, and new responsibilities—training students, taking call (gl), switching specialties. With each new step, a little voice may reappear: "Are you sure you can do this?"

The trick is not to wait until the voice disappears before you act. Instead, recognize it as a sign that you're growing. Ground yourself in what you do know, prepare as well as you can, and let experience slowly build a new kind of confidence—one that can coexist with humility.

I wish I had known how important it is to build a life outside the OR.

In the beginning, the work is so new and intense that it is easy to let it become your whole identity. You talk about cases at dinner, check the schedule on your day off, and feel restless when you are not under bright lights. On some level, it feels good to be needed and to have work that clearly matters.

But this job can take as much of you as you are willing to give. There will be stretches when you work long shifts, pick up extra call, or stay late for add-on cases. If you do not have anything outside of the hospital that feeds you—hobbies, friendships, rest—you risk burning out faster than you realize.

What many techs wish they had done earlier is set boundaries: saying no to one extra shift now and then, protecting one day a week for non-medical life, keeping at least one interest that has nothing to do with healthcare. The OR will keep spinning without you for a day. Your future self will be grateful you treated your whole life, not just your career, as something worth protecting.

Small story – "The year everything became about work."

It often starts with good intentions: helping out when the department is short, volunteering for overtime to pay off loans, saying yes whenever the charge nurse looks stressed. Months later, you realize you have not seen certain friends in weeks, and your world has shrunk to a hallway, a break room, and your bed. Only when you finally take a real vacation—or hit a wall and get sick—do you notice how tired you've been. Many techs look back and say, "I wish I had pulled back just a little sooner, before it took something drastic to make me stop."

I wish I had known that there are many ways to grow, not just "scrub forever."

When you picture your future, it might be hard to see beyond "work in the OR until I retire." In reality, this career has more branches than most people realize. Some techs specialize—cardiac, neuro (brain and spine) (gl), orthopedics, robotics (gl), labor and delivery. Some move into leadership roles as charge techs or supervisors. Some go into sterile processing management, education, or device company work. Some go back to school for nursing, physician assistant, anesthesiologist assistant, or other advanced roles.

You do not have to decide your whole path on day one. But it helps to know that you have options. When you realize, "I do not actually enjoy trauma nights, but I love robotics days," or, "I care more about teaching new techs than about being in the hardest rooms," that is not a failure. It is data you can use to steer.

The earlier you give yourself permission to imagine different futures, the less trapped you will feel when your interests or energy change.

I wish I had known that being "only the tech" is a lie—and that the work is bigger than you can see.

You may hear people say, half-joking, "We're just the techs." It can make you feel small, like you are replaceable, like the real work belongs to everyone else in the room. But look closely at what actually happens when surgery runs well.

You are the one who spots the contaminated sleeve, the missing needle, the wrong implant. You are the one who builds the surgeon's tools into a coherent, usable layout. You are the one who remembers that one surgeon hates a certain retractor or that this patient is latex-allergic (gl) and needs special supplies. You are often the quiet stability in the corner when tempers rise and everyone else is talking.

You will almost never be the one whose name is on the consent form. You will not be the person families ask for in the waiting room. But the care you give is woven into every safe outcome—every patient who wakes up without a retained sponge (gl), every wound that stays clean, every case that moves smoothly instead of chaotically. Many techs wish they had understood earlier that the invisibility of their role does not make it unimportant. It just means you have to be the one who remembers why it matters.

You cannot know everything before you start. Some lessons only land when you are the one standing at the field, gown tied, gloves on, heart pounding as the patient rolls in. But walking into this career with these truths already in your pocket makes a difference.

You can expect to feel lost at first and still keep going. You can prepare for the emotional weight as well as the technical steps. You can choose small habits that build a strong reputation. You can speak up, protect your own life outside of work, and allow your path to evolve. Most of all, you can remember that being a Surgical Technologist is not about being perfect—it is about showing up, case after case, with skill, honesty, and a willingness to keep learning, long after school is over.

Chapter 6
The Toll Booth

The Toll Booth — The Real Cost of Becoming a Surgical Technologist

Every healthcare career gives something meaningful to the world. Every healthcare career also takes something in return. That exchange — the physical, emotional, cognitive, and lifestyle cost of the role — is what we call the Toll Booth.

For Surgical Technologists, the toll is rarely obvious from the outside. Patients often meet the surgeon, the nurse, or the anesthesia provider, but the Surgical Technologist works quietly inside the sterile field, often unseen yet absolutely essential. The responsibility is real, the physical demand is steady, and the mental focus required across long procedures can be intense. Understanding this toll early does not discourage people from the profession; it protects them by helping them decide whether the environment truly fits their wiring.

The Physical Toll

Long surgical cases mean long hours standing in one position, often wearing heavy lead protection during imaging procedures or maintaining static postures while holding retractors. Back fatigue, shoulder strain, and foot discomfort can accumulate over time, particularly in specialties such as orthopedics, neurosurgery, and trauma. Surgical Technologists who learn early to prioritize footwear, posture, stretching, and strength conditioning often extend both their comfort and career longevity.

The Cognitive Toll

The operating room demands constant anticipation. Surgical Technologists must track instrument sequencing, surgeon preferences, sterile integrity, counts, equipment readiness, and procedural progression simultaneously. The mental load can feel manageable in routine cases but rises significantly during emergencies or complex surgeries. Individuals who naturally enjoy structured sequencing, precision, and sustained concentration often find this cognitive environment energizing rather than exhausting — a common pattern seen among certain **SCRUB*fits*™**, particularly those aligned with technical flow and procedural rhythm.

The Emotional Toll

Unlike some patient-facing roles, Surgical Technologists may have limited direct patient interaction, yet they still participate in life-changing procedures, traumatic injuries, and high-stakes surgical moments. Witnessing difficult outcomes, unexpected complications, or emotionally intense cases can carry weight even when the role requires composure and efficiency. Building recovery habits — debriefing with teammates, maintaining interests outside the hospital, and protecting personal downtime — becomes essential for long-term sustainability.

The Lifestyle Toll

Operating room schedules rarely follow perfect predictability. Early start times, add-on cases, emergency surgeries, call requirements, and occasional extended shifts can affect sleep routines, family schedules, and personal planning. Some Surgical Technologists thrive in this dynamic rhythm, while others prefer surgical centers or specialties with more predictable hours. Alignment often depends less on the profession itself and more on the specific surgical environment and team culture — another area where recognizing your **SCRUB*fits*™** alignment patterns can help guide smarter career decisions.

The Hidden Toll: Being the Invisible Professional

Many Surgical Technologists experience a quieter challenge — their work is highly skilled but not always visible to patients or the public. Recognition often comes internally from the surgical team rather than externally from those receiving care. For some professionals, this behind-the-scenes contribution feels deeply satisfying; for others, it can feel under-recognized. Understanding your own motivation style helps determine whether this dynamic feels comfortable or draining over time.

Why the Toll Booth Matters

The purpose of identifying the toll is not to measure difficulty; every healthcare role is demanding in different ways. The purpose is to help you ask a better question:

"Do the costs of this role match the strengths, preferences, and energy patterns I naturally bring?"

When the answer is yes, Surgical Technology becomes a career where skill, teamwork, and technical mastery can feel deeply rewarding. When the answer is no, the same environment can slowly erode energy even when performance remains strong. The most sustainable careers are not built on endurance alone; they are built on alignment — where your abilities, your temperament, and your daily work environment reinforce each other rather than compete.

Before moving forward, take a moment to reflect:

Which parts of the operating-room environment energize you most — the precision, the teamwork, the pace, the technology, the urgency, or the structured repetition?

Your answer offers one of the earliest signals of which Surgical Technologist pathways, specialties, and **SCRUB*fits*™** alignment patterns may fit you best.

Chapter 7
Side Hustles and Career Growth

There is a version of this career where you punch in, scrub (gl), punch out, watch TV, and repeat until retirement. For some people, that is enough. For others, the operating room (gl) is just the first doorway. You start as a Surgical Technologist (gl), but your skills can grow into extra income, new roles, and whole new careers if you are intentional about how you spend your time outside your main job.

You do not have to do everything at once. You do not have to hustle yourself into burnout. But it helps to know what is possible so you can make choices instead of drifting.

Side Hustle #1: Extra Shifts and Per Diem (gl) Work

The simplest side hustle is using the skills you already have for more hours or a higher rate. It is not glamorous, but it is real money.

You might:

• Pick up extra shifts through your own department when the schedule is short.

• Work as a per diem tech at another facility a few days a month.

• Join a local staffing pool that sends you to different ORs as needed.

This is realistic because you do not have to learn a new field; you are already trained. The onboarding is familiar, and per diem roles often pay more per hour than staff jobs. The trade-off is that you are still trading your body and energy for every dollar, and you can easily push yourself too far if you say yes every time someone is desperate for coverage.

The most sustainable way to use extra shifts is to give each dollar a job. You might decide that all per diem money goes toward debt, an emergency fund, or a specific savings goal. That way, you are not just working more for vague "extra" money; you are building something concrete and can scale back once those goals are met.

Side Hustle #2: Tutoring and Skills Coaching for Students

Every Surgical Technologist program is full of people who are overwhelmed and terrified of their first day in the OR. You are a few steps ahead of them. That gap is worth something.

You can:

• Offer one-on-one tutoring for anatomy (gl), instrumentation, and exam preparation.

• Run small skills sessions on how to set up a basic back

table, how to read preference cards, and how to avoid common contamination (gl) mistakes.

• Help students prepare for mock check-offs or certification (gl) exams.

This can happen in person if you live near a school, or online using video calls and case walk-throughs. You remember what it was like to feel lost, so you can translate OR language into plain, calm instructions. You will also learn whether teaching drains you or energizes you, which is useful information for later.

If you find that you truly enjoy helping newer people grow, this side hustle can grow into formal roles. You might become a clinical preceptor (gl), an orientation buddy for new hires, or even an instructor in a Surgical Technology program. You may eventually shift from holding retractors all day to holding a whiteboard marker, and that change starts with one student you help now.

Side Hustle #3: Creating Educational Content and Resources

You spend every shift in a world that most people never see. That experience can turn into content: writing, video, or tools that help others survive training and early practice.

You might:

• Write plain-language guides for new techs such as "First Day in the OR: What to Expect" or "Counts Without Panic."

• Make short videos explaining how to open sterile packs, how to pass instruments, or how to think through a simple case from setup to closure.

• Create digital resources like study planners, instrument flashcards, orientation trackers, or call (gl) shift debrief pages.

Your audience could be Surgical Technologist students, nursing students, or even family members trying to understand what you do. You have creative control and can build on your own schedule, during weeks when you actually have energy. The key is to protect patient privacy and never share anything that belongs to your employer.

Over time, these projects become a portfolio. If you later apply for educator, leadership, or industry roles, you can point to real things you have built, not just say, "I like teaching." This chapter of your career is not about going viral; it is about quietly building proof that you can explain complex work in a clear, grounded way.

Side Hustle #4: Health and Wellness Coaching for Healthcare Workers

If you are naturally drawn to routines, movement, and recovery, you might turn that interest into health coaching focused on people like you. Healthcare workers live in a different rhythm than nine-to-five jobs, and generic wellness advice often fails them.

You already understand:

• Long shifts on your feet.

• Chaotic meal times and break patterns.

• Stress that does not shut off when you swipe your badge out.

You might:

- Train as a certified health coach or personal trainer.
- Offer realistic programs for shift workers such as "Movement for people who stand all day" or "Simple meal planning for rotating shifts."
- Run small online groups for nurses, techs, and aides who want to feel better without quitting their jobs.

Because you live the same life they do, you have built-in credibility. The important part is to be honest with yourself. If you are already depleted, do not build a side hustle that drains the same muscles your main job uses. This kind of work makes the most sense if helping others with their health genuinely refills your emotional tank.

Down the line, you might still be in the OR part-time and coaching part-time, or you might eventually step fully into wellness work. Either way, you are using what you know about bodies and schedules in a way that serves both you and other people.

Side Hustle #5: Medical Product or Device Consulting on a Small Scale

Every new stapler, scope, or robot attachment is tested somewhere. Companies behind those tools need the perspective of people who actually use them in real cases. Your surgical experience gives you that perspective.

At a modest level, you might:

- Join feedback panels or surveys about new instruments or devices.

• Consult for a local company that is testing OR tools and needs clinician input.

• Help vendors understand how their instruments behave in real workflows instead of just in a lab.

You could be paid for occasional meetings, product trials, or structured interviews. You must be transparent with your employer about any conflict of interest (gl) and follow policy on outside work and confidentiality. The money from small consulting gigs might not replace a shift, but it introduces you to another side of healthcare.

Over time, you might find that you enjoy working with products and systems as much as with individual cases. That can lead into roles as a clinical specialist, device educator, or eventually into sales or project management for companies that support surgery.

Side Hustle #6: Travel Assignments as a Career Sampler

Travel contracts are not a part-time thing while you stay in your staff job. They are full-time for the length of the contract. But in the long arc of your working life, travel can function like a side path that gives you information and savings you would not get standing still.

If your life allows, you might:

• Take a travel contract in another city between longer stretches in staff roles.

• Use travel assignments to test different hospital cultures, specialties, and regions.

• Aim to bank a chunk of savings during one or two contracts and then return to a staff job with more flexibility and financial breathing room.

This kind of move often comes with higher hourly pay and stipends for housing, but less predictability. You learn how quickly you can adapt to new layouts, new surgeons, and new documentation systems. You also learn what kind of environment fits you best.

The point is not to become a permanent traveler unless you truly love that life. The point is to treat travel as a deliberate experiment: a temporary side road that gives you money and insight you can bring back to whatever long-term path you choose.

Side Hustle #7: Teaching OR Basics to Other Departments

Many people step into the OR from other parts of the hospital: radiology techs, students, environmental services, and float nurses. They are often nervous and do not fully understand sterile technique or OR culture. You can help close that gap.

You can:

• Create short in-service (gl) sessions about where to stand, how to move equipment without contaminating drapes, and what the sterile zones are.

• Help orient new staff who will be around the OR but not scrubbed in, like pre-op (gl), PACU (post-anesthesia care unit) (gl), or endoscopy colleagues.

• Offer to be a point person when units send staff down to observe surgeries or help with transports.

This might start informally with a small honorarium or educator pay from your hospital. Over time, it becomes evidence that you can design and deliver training, not just do the work yourself. That proof can support future moves into educator, coordinator, or management roles.

How this career can grow inside and beyond the OR

Side hustles are only part of the story. The other part is how you can grow within your main role. Not every Surgical Technologist wants to leave the OR; many just want more control over what they do there.

Common growth lanes include:

• Deep specialization in areas like cardiac, neuro, ortho, robotics (gl), or labor and delivery.

• Lead or senior tech roles that include mentoring and helping run the daily schedule.

• Educator roles that focus on training new techs, nurses, and students in OR skills and safety.

• Stepping into new professions such as nursing, anesthesia, or advanced practice, using your OR experience as a strong foundation.

The important thing is that you have more options than "scrub forever" or "quit." The skills you build in this role—anticipation, calm under pressure, communication, and technical fluency—are portable. Side hustles and small experiments let you test what you might want next without burning your current life down.

You do not have to know your entire future right now. You only need to be honest about what drains you, what sparks you, and what you are curious enough to try for a season. From there, you can let your career grow steadily instead of feeling like you are stuck in the same case list forever.

Chapter 8

Mini SCRUBfit™ Healthcare Career Assessment

Surgical Technologist Edition

Your Quick 1–10 Alignment Snapshot

This mini assessment helps you understand how naturally your wiring matches the pace, pressure, environment, and emotional rhythm of Surgical Technology.

Choose the answer that feels **most true for you**, most of the time.

Keep track of your points — you'll score yourself at the end.

How to Score Each Question

- **A = 1 point**
- **B = 0 points**

("A" represents alignment with core ST wiring; "B" represents partial alignment or mismatch.)

1. Pace Tolerance

A. I'm comfortable with fast-paced environments and quick transitions.

B. I prefer slow, quiet, low-stress spaces.

2. Pressure & Urgency

A. I stay steady when stakes are high or when surgeons move fast.

B. Pressure makes me feel rushed or overwhelmed.

3. Fine Motor Skills

A. I'm good with detailed, precise hand movements and tool handling.

B. I get frustrated with tiny, delicate tasks.

4. Anticipation

A. I naturally watch for cues and think one step ahead.

B. I prefer to wait for instructions.

5. Blood & Surgical Exposure

A. I can handle blood, tissue, and surgical visuals without shutting down.

B. These things bother me or make me uncomfortable.

6. Team Dynamics

A. I like tight teamwork, clear roles, and structured communication.

B. I prefer loose, flexible team environments where roles shift more freely.

7. Predictability vs. Chaos

A. I can handle sudden changes — new instruments, new steps, new needs.

B. Unexpected changes throw off my rhythm.

8. Physical Stamina

A. I can stand for long periods and stay focused for hours at a time.

B. I get fatigued easily or lose focus during long tasks.

9. Detail Orientation

A. I'm naturally detail-focused and notice small errors or contamination risks.

B. Details often slip by unless someone points them out.

10. Emotional Neutrality

A. I stay calm even when a surgeon is intense, frustrated, or demanding.

B. Emotional intensity sticks with me or impacts my performance.

Now Add Your Points

Count 1 point for every **A** you chose.

Your total score (0–10) is your **SCRUBfit™ Surgical Technologist Alignment Score.**

Your SCRUBfit™ Surgical Technologist Fit Score

9–10 Points: Strong Alignment

You are highly aligned with the demands, pace, and emotional tone of Surgical Technology.

Expect:

• Fast mastery

• High confidence

• Strong specialty potential (orthopedics, trauma, neuro, robotics)

• Lower burnout risk

• Strong team fit in most OR environments

You're wired for the OR.

7–8 Points: Good Alignment

You're a solid fit for Surgical Technology with strengths in many core areas.

Expect:

• Good adaptability

• Strong teamwork potential

• Comfort in a wide variety of specialties

• Growth through experience and repetition

You will thrive with the right team and environment.

5–6 Points: Moderate Alignment

You may enjoy parts of ST work but struggle in others.

Expect:

- Better fit in predictable, lower-acuity specialties (ENT, plastics, OB/GYN, general)
- Strong need for supportive team dynamics
- Possible challenges with high-intensity rooms

You can still succeed — but alignment varies by specialty.

3–4 Points: Low Alignment

There's some fit, but not with fast or complex OR environments.

Expect:

- Best fit in calmer service lines or ancillary surgical roles
- Higher burnout risk in fast rooms (ortho, trauma, neuro)

You may enjoy the surgical world—but perhaps not the heart of the OR itself.

0–2 Points: Minimal Alignment

Your natural wiring does not match the core demands of Surgical Technology.

Expect:

- High stress in fast-paced surgical rooms
- Fatigue from long cases or intense surgeons
- Better alignment in patient-facing or non-OR technical roles

This doesn't mean healthcare isn't right for you — just that *another* **SCRUB*fit*™** *category* may be a better long-term fit.

Why This Mini Assessment Works So Well

It mirrors your Alignment Theory:

Identity → Pace → Environment → Practice

And it makes the reader feel:

- Understood
- Supported
- Seen
- Empowered
- Engaged with your brand

And it gives everyone — students, new grads, career changers, and experienced STs — a **quick clarity snapshot** they can use immediately.

It's perfect for ScrubTales™.

Chapter 9

What Your Fit Score Really Means for Your Future

Your Fit Score isn't a grade, a judgment, or a prediction of success.

It's a snapshot of alignment — how naturally your wiring, pace preferences, and emotional patterns match the environment of Surgical Technology.

Alignment is not about talent alone.

It's about fit.

When the environment matches who you are, confidence grows, skill develops quickly, and the work feels meaningful.

When it doesn't, the job feels heavier than it should — even for talented people.

This page helps you interpret what your score says about your best next steps.

If You Scored 9–10: Strong Alignment

You're wired for the OR (gl) pace, pressure, and precision.

This career won't just be a match — it will likely feel energizing.

You may excel in:

- Orthopedics
- Trauma
- Neuro (gl)
- Spine (gl)
- Cardiothoracic (gl)
- High-volume general surgery
- Robotics (gl)

Your biggest opportunities:

- Early specialty training
- Strong surgeon partnerships
- Rapid advancement into advanced service lines
- Leadership pathways within surgical services

Your biggest caution:

- Overcommitting because the OR (gl) feels natural — protect your boundaries.

If You Scored 7–8: Good Alignment

You are a strong fit for Surgical Technology and will thrive with repetition and experience.

You may excel in:

- Laparoscopy (gl)
- General surgery
- OB/GYN (gl)
- Urology (gl)
- ENT (gl)
- Multi-service float pools (gl)

Your biggest opportunities:

- Becoming a highly adaptable, cross-trained ST (gl)
- Finding a team culture that supports communication
- Growing steadily into more complex rooms

Your biggest caution:

- Avoid rooms that stay in crisis-mode all day until you feel ready.

If You Scored 5–6: Moderate Alignment

You have the wiring to succeed in this field — but your alignment depends on the type of OR (gl) and the type of specialty.

You may excel in:

- Predictable service lines
- Lower-acuity (gl) rooms
- Calm, well-structured teams

You may want to avoid:

- High-intensity rooms early in your career
- Trauma-heavy or neuro-heavy roles
- Surgeons with aggressive communication styles

Your biggest opportunities:

- Finding the right specialty fit
- Developing confidence through repetition
- Building routine before adding complexity

Many great Surgical Technologists fall right in this range.

If You Scored 3–4: Low Alignment

You can still do the work, but the OR (gl) may feel heavier or more draining for you.

You may prefer:

- Endoscopy (gl)
- Central sterile (gl)
- Clinic-based surgical support
- Minor procedure rooms
- Eye surgery centers
- Outpatient plastics

These environments offer:

- Predictability
- Lower stress
- Shorter cases

- Familiar teams

Your biggest opportunities:

- Choosing environments that protect your energy
- Building a surgical career that fits your strengths

Your biggest caution:

- Don't force yourself into trauma or ortho if your wiring says otherwise.

If You Scored 0–2: Minimal Alignment

Your strengths may lie outside the main OR (gl) — and that's not a weakness.

You may prefer:

- Patient-facing roles
- Technical but low-stress environments
- Diagnostic roles
- Front-end or back-end surgical support
- Healthcare pathways with slower pace and different sensory demands

Examples:

- Sterile processing (gl)
- Medical imaging (gl)
- Ambulatory (gl) surgical support
- Clinic procedure assisting

- Lab or pathology tech roles (gl)

Your biggest opportunities:

- A career pivot that honors your strengths
- Exploring other **SCRUB*fit*™** categories
- Using this insight to choose a role where you thrive

Remember:

This score doesn't say you can't, it simply tells you where the work will feel most natural and sustainable.

Why Alignment Matters in the OR

The OR (gl) is demanding — physically, mentally, emotionally, and socially.

When your wiring matches the environment, you grow.

When it clashes, you grind.

Your score shows you:

- Where the OR (gl) will bring out your best
- Where you may struggle
- Where burnout risk is highest
- Where confidence will build fastest
- Where mastery is most attainable
- Where you will feel the most "you"

This is the heart of **SCRUB*fit*™**:

Identity × Pace × Environment × Practice

Everything feels easier when those four align.

Your Next Step

Now that you know your Fit Score, keep it in mind as you read the 15 Day-In-The-Life vignettes. Pay attention to the days that:

- Feel energizing
- Sound like "your pace"
- Make you feel excited or grounded
- Match your internal rhythm

Those are the rooms where you will thrive.

This is just the beginning of your alignment journey — but it's a powerful first step.

Chapter 10

Alignment and Reflection

There is the job on paper, and then there is the job in your body. One is a list of duties and shifts. The other is the way your chest feels when the alarm goes off before sunrise, the way your shoulders feel when you see tomorrow's schedule, the way your mind feels when you walk out into the dark parking lot.

Alignment (gl) is about whether those two versions of the job line up with who you are and the life you actually want.

You do not have to guess with perfect accuracy what you will want fifteen years from now. You do not have to promise that you will love every moment of this work. What you can do is pay attention to what lights you up, what drains you, and which signals you have been quietly ignoring. Reflection is how you listen to those signals on purpose instead of letting them whisper in the background.

Use the prompts below like a private debrief with yourself. You can write your answers, type them into a notes app, record them as voice memos, or just think through them during a quiet walk. The format does not matter. Your honesty does.

What lit you up

• Think back to the last time you felt genuinely energized in a clinical (gl), lab, or healthcare setting. What were you doing in that moment? Who else was there, and what was your role?

• When you imagine yourself fully inside this career, which specific moments give you a small spark of "I want that"? Is it setting up a space, being part of a tight team, mastering a technical skill, or something else?

• Recall a day when time passed quickly because you were deeply focused. What kind of tasks were you doing? Moving fast between tasks, working on one complex problem, helping someone understand something, organizing chaos?

• Notice any times you felt quietly proud, even if no one else noticed. What were you doing, and what did that say about what matters to you?

What gave you dread

• Think about a time you felt a real pit in your stomach before a shift, a class, or a clinical day. What exactly were you dreading—the people, the pace, the unpredictability, the physical strain, the emotional load?

• When you picture a typical week in this career, what parts make you tense up? Early alarms, long days on your feet, last-minute changes, being around strong emotions, or something else?

• Imagine you have been in this role for one year. It is Sunday night. What do you feel when you think about Monday: "let's go," "I can get through it," or "I cannot keep doing this"?

• Be specific. "I dread being tired" is different from "I dread not having control over my schedule" or "I dread being snapped at in public." Each one points to a different kind of misalignment.

What felt meaningful

• Think about a moment in any job or experience where you felt, "This matters." What were you doing, and who did it help?

• When you imagine yourself in this path, what kind of impact feels most meaningful: protecting safety, supporting patients and families, keeping systems organized, teaching others, or something else?

• If you could only keep one part of the work—the technical challenge, the people, the sense of purpose, the stability, the paycheck—which one would you choose, and why?

• Ask yourself: does this career give me a realistic path to the kind of meaning I care about, or am I hoping it will magically feel meaningful because it is in healthcare?

What your body is telling you

• How does your body feel after a physically demanding day: tired-but-okay, wrung out, or strangely calm? Which parts complain the loudest—feet, back, neck, head?

• How do early mornings, irregular meals, and long stretches of focus land in your system? Do you bounce back with a single good night's sleep, or does it take days to feel normal again?

• What does "enough rest" look like for you in a normal week? Can you see any version of this career where that kind of rest happens more often than not?

• When you think about doing this work for years, does your body feel more like it is bracing or more like it is settling into something it can grow stronger in?

Your life outside of work

• Think about the people who matter most to you. How do you imagine a healthcare schedule affecting your time, attention, and patience with them?

• Do you recharge more with quiet alone time, with social time, or with doing something physical? Where would that fit around this kind of work?

• When you picture your life five years from now, what do you want your average week to look like? How many evenings at home, how many days off in a row, how much mental space for interests outside of healthcare?

• Can you imagine this career bending toward that picture with some realistic trade-offs, or does it feel like you would be building a life around surviving work and recovering from it?

The sentence you do not want to say out loud

• Finish this sentence honestly: "Right now, I am moving toward this career mostly because..."

• Then finish this one: "If I did not have to impress or please anyone else, I would secretly want to..."

• Notice the gap—if there is one—between those two answers. That gap is where misalignment often hides.

You do not owe anyone a specific answer after this reflection. You do owe yourself honesty. Alignment is not about finding a "perfect" career with no stress. It is about choosing a path where the stress you take on feels worth it to you, for reasons that actually belong to you and not to anyone else.

Chapter 11

The 101™ Q&A on Becoming a Surgical Technologist

Q1. What does a Surgical Technologist actually *do* in the operating room?

A Surgical Technologist is the quiet architect of the operating room — the person who builds the sterile universe in which surgery can safely happen. Before the surgeon ever steps into the room, you've already begun shaping the entire environment: pulling cases, checking trays, inspecting instruments for damage, verifying sterility indicators, and making sure everything the surgeon might need is accounted for. It's more than preparation — it's prediction. You walk through the procedure in your mind before anyone else has even arrived.

Once the patient enters, your role deepens. You help position them, assist with prepping and draping, and build the sterile field layer by layer with disciplined precision. During the case itself, you become the surgeon's right hand — passing instruments with speed and accuracy, anticipating the next step before it's spoken, maintaining vigilance over the sterile field, and adjusting to changes in real time. Your eyes are everywhere: the Mayo stand, the back table, the wound, the hands moving around the field, the instruments returning for cleaning, the counts, the sutures, the rhythm of the room.

And then there's the part no one teaches with words — the emotional intelligence. You read a surgeon's silence. You feel a shift in the room's pace. You listen not just to what's said but to what *isn't*. You steady the room when tension rises and keep the entire team anchored when complications appear.

A Surgical Technologist is not an assistant to surgery — you are a guardian of patient safety, a conductor of flow, and an expert in surgical choreography. Without you, there is no sterile field, no efficient sequence, no protected space for the surgeon to operate. You make the OR possible.

Q2. Is being a Surgical Technologist the same as being a scrub tech?

Yes — and no. The term "scrub tech" is the informal name that stuck because it describes one of your primary responsibilities: scrubbing in and maintaining the sterile field. But "Surgical Technologist" is the full, formal, professional title that encompasses far more than just handing instruments across a draped table.

A scrub tech focuses on the direct, hands-on aspects of surgery: gowning, gloving, setting up sterile instrumentation, and working at the surgeon's side. But a Surgical Technologist operates across the entire surgical continuum. Before the incision, you're a planner, analyst, and architect. You pull cases, evaluate supplies, ensure sterility, inspect instruments, and coordinate with circulating nurses to prepare the room for a procedure that may not even begin for another hour. Your preparation defines the flow of the entire case.

During the operation, you are not just passing instruments — you're orchestrating them. You maintain the sterile field, anticipate the surgeon's moves, protect the patient's safety, and help drive the tempo of the room. Your hands and the surgeon's hands become synced through repetition, intuition, and trust.

After the case, you transform again: breaking down the field, cleaning instruments, returning equipment, preparing specialized items for reprocessing, and resetting the room for the next procedure. The scrub technician role explains *what your hands do*, but the Surgical Technologist title reflects *what your brain does*. You manage details, protect sterility, support the surgical team, and keep the rhythm of a high-stakes environment moving from case to case without collapse.

So yes — "scrub tech" is accurate, but it's incomplete. When you step into the profession, you're stepping into a role with depth, responsibility, and a level of technical precision that deserves its full title: **Surgical Technologist.**

Q3. How do Surgical Technologists keep patients safe if they never speak to them?

It's one of the most beautiful paradoxes of the profession: the patient rarely sees you. They don't know your name, don't see your face behind the mask, don't remember you because they're sedated by the time you truly enter their story — yet you play one of the most crucial roles in protecting them.

Your safety work begins long before the patient arrives. Every instrument you inspect, every tray you open, every piece of equipment you test contributes to preventing errors and complications. A cracked instrument, a missing screw, a compromised wrapper — these are not minor details. They are potential surgical disasters avoided because of your vigilance.

When the patient enters, your presence becomes quieter but more essential. You ensure the sterile field is uncompromised — that no sleeve brushes too close, no drape shifts, no instrument crosses a boundary that could put the patient at risk. Your eyes stay on the field even when your hands are busy. You anticipate needs before they become urgent. If contamination occurs, you are often the first to see it, acknowledge it, and correct it.

During surgery, your ability to pass instruments efficiently isn't just about speed — it's about minimizing open time. The shorter the procedure, the lower the complication risk. Your precision reduces hesitation, confusion, or unnecessary movement. You maintain counts that prevent retained surgical items, one of the most serious safety consequences in the OR.

And after the case, your work continues. Safe handling of instruments, verifying counts, protecting sharps, ensuring supplies move to decontamination properly — all of this prevents downstream errors.

You may not speak to the patient, but you protect them at every step. They may never see you, but your work will follow them for the rest of their life — in the scar that healed without infection, in the joint that moves freely again, in the operation that ended as simply as it began.

Q4. What is the hardest part of being a Surgical Technologist?

The hardest part isn't the long hours, the physical demands, the early mornings, or even the pressure of standing inches from the surgical site during moments of crisis — though all of that is real. The hardest part is something quieter, something more internal: carrying the emotional responsibility of perfection in a world where mistakes can have consequences.

Unlike other roles where errors can be corrected later, Surgical Technologists work in a world where seconds matter, sterility is absolute, and anticipation is not a luxury — it's survival. You must not only know the procedure; you must *predict* it. You must read the surgeon's tone, understand the rhythm of the room, sense subtle shifts in tension, and stay ahead without being asked.

You must stay calm when the unexpected happens — when bleeding worsens, when an instrument breaks, when a surgeon's voice tightens, when a room full of people suddenly moves as if the air has changed temperature. Your heartbeat must not betray you. Your hands must not hesitate. You learn to breathe differently in the OR — deeper, steadier, controlled.

There is also the emotional distance. You often do not know the patient's story. You do not get closure. You may never learn whether the operation saved their life or merely bought time. You give everything — your strength, your focus, your vigilance — and then you reset the room, open a new tray, and begin again for someone else whose story will also remain incomplete.

And yet, the hardest part is also what makes the profession meaningful. The pressure exists because what you do matters. You train for this. You grow into this. You learn to carry the weight not as a burden but as a calling — and the day you realize you can hold it without fear is the day you become a true Surgical Technologist.

Q5. How does a Surgical Technologist learn to anticipate the surgeon's needs?

Anticipation is a skill you won't fully understand until you live inside an OR long enough for your brain to map the flow of a procedure like choreography. At first, anticipation feels impossible — like trying to guess the next line in a song you've never heard before. But over time, repetition, pattern recognition, and observation transform you.

You begin by learning the anatomy of the procedure: the steps, the order, the common variations. But anatomy alone isn't enough — anticipation requires understanding *why* the surgeon chooses each move. You start listening not just with your ears but with your eyes. You watch their posture, their hand positions, the way their voice shifts, the tiny hesitation before they reach. Surgeons have signatures just like musicians.

Eventually, you no longer pass an instrument because they ask — you pass it because you feel the moment arrive. You recognize the micro-pause before the next step. You sense the tension that means a clamp is needed, the angle of a wrist that predicts a retractor shift, the subtle change in lighting that signals suction.

And then something remarkable happens: your brain begins running a quiet simulation in the background. Three steps ahead. Five. Seven. You know when to prepare the next instrument, when to load a suture, when to start opening a new pack.

Anticipation is trust in motion. It tells the surgeon, *"You are not alone. I am with you. I know this procedure too."*

This is why Surgical Technologists are not just assistants — they are partners in the choreography of surgery. Anticipation is not magic. It is mastery born of presence, repetition, observation, humility, and finally — confidence.

Q6. What do Surgical Technologists need to know about instruments that most people never think about?

Most people think an instrument is just a tool. But to a Surgical Technologist, each instrument is a character with its own personality, function, and quirks — and your job is to know them intimately. You learn the weight of a Kelly clamp by feel alone. You memorize the sound a misaligned rongeur makes when it clicks incorrectly. You learn that some needle drivers loosen with age and need earlier maintenance. Instruments have temperaments, and you become fluent in their language.

You must also understand instrument *sequencing*: not just what tool to hand, but when and why. A surgeon doesn't want "a clamp"; they want *the specific clamp that fits the tissue, the vector of force, and the next step.* You recognize whether the case needs a long or short version, curved or straight, heavy or delicate, toothed or smooth.

Then there's the responsibility of safety. A cracked instrument can cause catastrophic complications. A dull blade can tear instead of cut. A broken tip can disappear into a cavity. You learn to examine everything — springs, hinges, serrations, jaws, alignment — because your patient's life depends on your ability to detect what most would ignore.

You also manage tray organization. The back table isn't random — it's a landscape of instincts. The most frequently used instruments sit closest. Rare items sit at angles you can reach without looking. The Mayo stand becomes an extension of your hands.

What most people never understand is this: Surgical instruments are not passive objects. They are part of a living system. And you — with your trained eyes, steady hands, and disciplined awareness — are the keeper of that system.

Q7. What is the role of a Surgical Technologist during emergency surgery?

Emergency surgery is where a Surgical Technologist truly becomes indispensable. When a trauma rolls in, the room transforms — alarms, footsteps, urgency layered into every voice. There is no script. No warm-up. No time to plan. And yet, you must bring order into chaos.

Your first job is to prepare the room faster than anyone else can think. You pull the necessary trays, open essential supplies, check instruments for immediate use, and set the sterile field with the speed of someone who knows minutes matter. Surgeons are coming. Anesthesiology is preparing. The patient may be crashing. You build a battlefield in seconds.

During the operation, your responsibilities intensify. Emergencies don't unfold neatly — they twist. Bleeding worsens. Anatomy distorts. Instruments must arrive instantly, not eventually. You pass retractors, suction, clamps, vascular instruments, emergency sutures, and sponges almost in a blur. You stay vigilant with counts even when the pace is overwhelming, because safety cannot collapse just because the situation is frightening.

Your emotional regulation becomes your superpower. While everyone else escalates, you descend into calm. Your breathing slows. Your eyes sharpen. You become the quiet center of the storm — the one person who does not panic. Surgeons feel your steadiness. Nurses rely on your order. The entire room anchors to your composure.

After the case, you may never know what happened to the patient. Trauma is a world of beginnings, not endings. But you will know this: when the lights were bright and the pressure was high, you stood exactly where you needed to be — steady, skilled, unshaken.

Q8. How do Surgical Technologists deal with difficult surgeons?

Surgical Technologists work in a world where personalities range from gentle mentors to intense perfectionists — and sometimes, the surgeon standing across from you is someone who pushes hard, speaks sharply, or expects you to anticipate their needs flawlessly. You learn quickly that the OR is a pressure cooker for everyone—surgeons included—and that difficult behavior often reflects stress, not malice.

The first skill you develop is emotional neutrality. You do not personalize comments spoken in urgency. You recognize that surgeons often speak in shorthand under pressure, and their tone reflects the stakes of the procedure, not the value of the people in the room. You become comfortable letting intensity pass through you rather than hitting you.

Next, you learn the language of preference. Difficult surgeons are often predictable if you study them. You learn their instrument sequence, their pet peeves, their timing. You observe how they like their sutures cut, how they angle retractors, when they want suction without asking, when they expect silence. Predictability turns confrontation into teamwork.

You also learn to communicate professionally. "I hear you," "I've got it," or "It's coming now" diffuse tension without escalating the moment. After the case, if something genuinely needs discussion, you bring it up calmly — or your charge tech does.

Most importantly, you discover that difficult surgeons often transform once they trust you. The ones who push the hardest sometimes become your greatest allies when they see your consistency, your anticipation, your resilience.

Over time, you develop a thick skin, a soft heart, and an unshakeable sense of purpose:

You're not there to take things personally.

You're there to protect the patient.

And nothing — not tension, not tone, not ego — comes before that.

Q9. What is the most rewarding part of being a Surgical Technologist?

It's not the instruments, though you'll come to love them.

It's not the rhythm, though the flow of surgery is unlike anything else.

It's not even the trust you build with surgeons, though that becomes a profound professional bond.

The most rewarding part is something quieter:

the way your presence helps someone return to their life.

You may never see the patient awake. You may never hear their voice or learn their story. But you know that because of your preparation — your sterile field, your counts, your anticipation, your vigilance — a mother will go home to her children again, a grandparent will walk pain-free again, a student will return to school, a worker will resume their livelihood, a life interrupted will be restored.

You will watch organs repaired, bones realigned, tumors removed, bleeding stopped, hope restored — all without ever receiving recognition from the patient themselves. The reward is knowing you made it possible without needing applause.

There is also a personal transformation. As you grow, you discover that you are capable of more strength, focus, and resilience than you ever imagined. You learn to stay steady in situations others could not endure. You learn to think deeply while moving quickly. You learn to be the calm that others lean on.

You realize your work matters not because anyone sees it, but because **it must be done perfectly to keep someone alive.**

And that kind of meaning doesn't fade.

It grows.

Q10. How does a Surgical Technologist handle the pressure when things go wrong?

When things go wrong in the OR — bleeding escalates, anatomy surprises, equipment fails, tension spikes — the Surgical Technologist becomes one of the most critical stabilizing forces in the room. You don't have the luxury of panic. You have a patient on the table and a surgeon who needs your hands steady and your mind sharp.

You draw from training first. Every program, every rotation, every simulation teaches you one core truth: fall back on your steps. Protect the sterile field. Get the right instrument. Keep the counts accurate. Move with purpose, not speed. Anchor yourself in the basics.

Then, experience takes over. You learn the subtle cues of a deteriorating situation — the way a surgeon's voice tightens, the shift in suction rhythm, the sudden call for vascular instruments, the way anesthesia straightens in their chair. Your heart may spike for a moment, but your breathing slows, your vision narrows, and your hands move almost automatically to prepare for what comes next.

Emotionally, you rely on compartmentalization — not avoidance, but timing. You tell your brain: *This fear belongs later. Not now.*

Later may be the locker room. Or your car. Or your shower. But not the sterile field.

Afterward, you debrief. You replay the moment. You ask what could have been done differently. You integrate the lessons into your muscle memory so the next emergency catches you wiser, not weaker.

Handling pressure isn't about being unafraid.

It's about staying functional inside the fear —

and knowing the patient relies on that.

Q11. How do Surgical Technologists prepare for a procedure they've never seen before?

Walking into a case you've never seen feels like stepping into a darkened theater moments before the play begins — you don't know the lines, the pacing, the cues, or the emotional temperature yet. But you're still a part of the performance, and preparation is how you light your way.

First, you study the procedure. Most facilities maintain preference cards, procedural guides, or digital case libraries. You look up the sequence, critical steps, common variations, and instruments required. Then, you ask the circulating nurse or experienced techs for insight: "What does Dr. ___ do differently in this case?" The subtleties — not the big steps — are what define a smooth flow.

Next, you examine the trays meticulously. Unfamiliar cases may come with specialized sets, so you take extra time to orient yourself. You handle the instruments one by one, learning their weight and purpose. If something seems unclear, you ask before the incision, never during.

During setup, you rehearse quietly in your mind: incision → exposure → dissection → correction → closure. You imagine the order the surgeon might request instruments. This mental run-through becomes your invisible safety net.

When the case begins, humility becomes your biggest asset. You stay observant, calm, and responsive. You watch the surgeon's body language. You listen for patterns. You ask clarifying questions early, not late. And as the case progresses, you begin to anticipate naturally — the steps unfold, and you fall into rhythm.

By the end, you realize something important: unfamiliar does not mean unprepared. Every Surgical Technologist learns to thrive in the unknown not by memorizing every procedure but by mastering the mindset of curiosity, composure, and adaptability.

This is how you grow your skill set — one unfamiliar case at a time.

Q12. How do Surgical Technologists stay calm in high-stress operating rooms?

Calm isn't something you're born with — it's something the OR teaches you. The first time a surgeon's tone sharpens, or a complication unfolds, or the room vibrates with urgency, your heart may race. But over time, calm becomes your professional identity.

The secret is **controlled focus**. When a stressful moment hits — bleeding spikes, vital signs drop, an unexpected anatomy variation appears — you narrow your focus to what you can control: your hands, your instruments, your field. You anchor your attention to the sterile field like it's the center of gravity in a storm.

Another strategy is **breath training**. Many techs swear by a slow inhale through the nose, a three-second hold, and a gentle exhale through the mouth. It's subtle, invisible under your mask, and instantly steadies your hands.

You also learn to trust your training. Emergencies feel overwhelming until you've lived through enough of them to recognize patterns. You know when to pass vascular clamps, when to move suction closer, when to prep sponges for rapid counts, and when to simply stand still and steady.

Emotional distance helps too. You don't detach from the patient — you detach from panic. You treat chaos as a cue, not a threat. "Something is happening. My role matters even more now."

Most importantly, you lean on your team. A calm anesthesia provider, a seasoned circulator, a supportive surgeon — their steadiness becomes contagious. Over time, *you* become the steady one others rely on.

Calm isn't the absence of fear — it's the mastery of it. And Surgical Technologists become calm because the OR demands it, shapes it, and eventually engraves it into who you are.

Q13. How much medical knowledge does a Surgical Technologist actually need?

A Surgical Technologist is not just a technical assistant — you are a hybrid of anatomist, technician, safety officer, and procedural strategist. Your medical knowledge must be deep enough to make you functional, safe, and proactive in one of the most complex environments in healthcare.

You need a strong grasp of **anatomy**: organs, vessels, layers of tissue, musculoskeletal landmarks, and surgical planes. When a surgeon asks for a specific retractor, they assume you understand the anatomy they're exposing. When they say "we're close to the nerve," you must know which nerve, where it runs, and what instrument protects it.

You must understand **surgical pathology** — why the procedure is being done. Removing a gallbladder for inflammation differs significantly from removing one due to cancer. Repairing a fracture differs from revising a failed orthopedic implant. Pathology influences instruments, timing, and flow.

You also need working knowledge of **pharmacology**, especially local anesthetics, irrigation solutions, and medications frequently used in the sterile field.

And then there's **microbiology**, one of the pillars of your profession. Understanding how bacteria spread, how contamination occurs, and how sterility fails is foundational. The sterile field isn't just a concept — it's a set of microbiological truths that your hands enforce.

You don't need to diagnose or prescribe, but you need to think clinically. You need to understand why a step matters, not just how to do it.

Your knowledge doesn't make you a doctor — it makes you a Surgical Technologist.

And that distinction matters.

Q14. What is it like working with anesthesia providers in the OR?

Anesthesia is the quiet heartbeat of the operating room — the presence behind the drape ensuring the patient remains safe, stable, and unaware. As a Surgical Technologist, your relationship with anesthesia is collaborative, respectful, and essential.

You begin before the incision. As you prepare your field, you listen for anesthesia's needs: airway equipment, IV access, medication administration, positioning requests. You coordinate with them to ensure the patient is placed safely and comfortably before sterile drapes cover them.

During the case, anesthesia monitors the patient's vitals, adjusts medications, manages the airway, and catches subtle changes that signal developing complications. You remain aware of anesthesia even while working at the sterile field. If they call out, "Suction!" during intubation or, "Pause — pressure dropping," you respond instantly, adjusting your actions to support the patient.

Communication is concise and respectful. You don't shout across the field — you speak with clarity and intention. "We're about to turn the bed," "Passing heavy retractors," or "Suction coming under the drape" are simple phrases that keep anesthesia aligned with your movements.

Anesthesia providers often appreciate Surgical Technologists more than anyone realizes. You bring structure and predictability to a room where they manage the most unpredictable part of surgery — the human body.

When the case ends, you watch the patient wake, listen to anesthesia assess airway safety, and prepare for transfer. You help position lines, secure drapes, and maintain sterility during the transition.

Working with anesthesia teaches you teamwork at the deepest level — two disciplines, one patient, one outcome.

Q15. What does a "smooth case" look like for a Surgical Technologist?

A smooth case feels like music — each person hitting their cues, each step flowing seamlessly into the next, each movement predictable yet precise. For a Surgical Technologist, this is what harmony in the OR looks like.

It begins with preparation. Your trays arrive intact, your instruments pass inspection, and your sterile field builds cleanly. The room is calm, stocked, and ready before the surgeon enters. The circulating nurse trusts your setup; anesthesia is aligned; the patient is positioned flawlessly.

Once the incision begins, the choreography takes over. You pass instruments without hesitation. The surgeon reaches out, and your hand meets theirs at the perfect moment. The field stays pristine. Suction, retraction, cutting, suturing — everything flows in an unbroken rhythm. Even the unexpected becomes manageable because you've anticipated three steps ahead.

Counts are accurate. Instruments return clean. Nothing goes missing. Sponges stack neatly. The back table remains organized even as the case progresses.

The best smooth cases are silent symphonies — not because no one speaks, but because communication is purposeful, efficient, and respectful. You don't hear yelling. You hear teamwork.

When closure begins, everything feels lighter. You prepare sutures before being asked. You load needles precisely. You transition to dressings with an effortless confidence that makes the room feel balanced.

After the final count and dressing, you break down quickly and cleanly. The surgeon leaves satisfied. The nurse thanks you. The next case begins with clarity instead of chaos.

A smooth case is not just a technical success — it is a moment of pride. It is the proof that you've mastered not only the steps but the spirit of the OR.

Q16. How do Surgical Technologists stay physically healthy in such a demanding job?

The OR is a physically intense workplace. You stand for hours, lean over tables, reposition patients, lift trays, and operate in environments that demand physical endurance and stability. Staying healthy isn't optional — it's survival.

First, posture becomes your religion. You learn to shift your weight subtly, align your spine, and avoid locking your knees. Many techs develop "OR stances" — micro-adjusted positions that keep strain off your lower back.

Stretching is essential. Whether it's a quick hamstring stretch during turnover or a shoulder roll before gowning, these small movements prevent long-term injuries. Many techs stretch religiously before and after shifts.

Strength training helps too. You don't need to be a bodybuilder, but a strong core and back protect you from injury when lifting trays or assisting with patient positioning. Even 10 minutes of strength work a day makes a difference.

Ergonomics become part of your mindset. You adjust table heights to match the surgeon, not your discomfort. You reposition steps to prevent awkward reaching. You ask for help lifting heavy trays — pride never heals a back injury.

Hydration and nutrition matter more than most new techs realize. Hot OR lamps and long cases dehydrate you quickly. Smart techs drink water before scrubbing in and eat protein-heavy snacks between cases.

Finally, rest is sacred. The OR is not kind to exhausted bodies. Sleep restores your reflexes, attention, and emotional composure.

A healthy Surgical Technologist is not just physically strong — they're strategic, aware, and proactive about protecting the body that carries them through a demanding and remarkable career.

Q17. What is the learning curve like during clinical rotations?

Clinical rotations introduce you to the real OR — the pace, the personalities, the pressure, the beauty, and the controlled chaos. The learning curve is steep, but it's also one of the most rewarding phases of your journey.

In the beginning, everything feels foreign. You're learning new instruments, memorizing tray names, figuring out where supplies live, and trying to understand the unspoken rules of OR culture. Surgeons speak fast. Techs move fast. Everyone seems to know what's happening except you.

Then something shifts. After a few weeks, you begin recognizing instruments by sight and then by feel. You observe procedures enough times that sequences stop being mysteries and start becoming patterns. You learn when to step forward and when to step back. Your voice grows steadier.

Your confidence builds as you scrub into more cases. You learn aseptic technique at a level no classroom can teach. You practice gowning and gloving until it's second nature. You develop subtle muscle memory — how to position a Mayo stand, how to set up a back table, how to pass a knife safely, how to protect the sterile field when the situation becomes crowded or tense.

By the end of your rotations, you may not feel like an expert, but you feel like you belong. The OR no longer intimidates you — it challenges you.

The learning curve is steep, but every step teaches you something essential: that growth happens at the edge of discomfort. And by graduation, you've earned the right to call yourself a Surgical Technologist-in-training, ready for the next level.

Q18. How do you know whether you're improving as a Surgical Technologist?

Improvement isn't always loud. It doesn't arrive with applause or announcements. In the OR, progress shows up in small, meaningful ways — ways only you and the people who work beside you can see.

You know you're improving when your setup becomes faster and more intuitive. You no longer second-guess tray placement or hesitate when choosing instruments. You move with intention instead of uncertainty.

You know you're improving when surgeons stop narrating every step because they trust you to anticipate what comes next. They reach out — and your hand is already there, offering exactly what they need.

You know you're improving when the circulating nurse says, "Thanks for being so organized," or "I love working with you." These quiet acknowledgments mean your teamwork is showing.

You know you're improving when your counts are clean, accurate, and confident — not rushed or fearful.

You know you're improving when you stop panicking during unexpected moments. When an instrument malfunctions, bleeding increases, or a surgeon changes the plan, you remain composed.

You know you're improving when you start mentoring newer students — even if you still feel like a beginner yourself. Teaching reveals how much you've truly learned.

And eventually, you know you're improving when the OR becomes a place you understand rather than a place you endure. The noise becomes music. The pace becomes rhythm. The pressure becomes clarity.

Improvement isn't measured in perfection. It's measured in presence.

And if you're showing up, learning, adjusting, and caring — you're improving.

Q19. Do Surgical Technologists get emotionally attached to the cases they participate in?

You might think that a job where the patient is asleep and unseen would keep emotions at a distance — but the opposite is often true. Surgical Technologists see some of the most vulnerable, heroic, heartbreaking, and hopeful moments in medicine.

You may never speak to most patients, but you witness their stories through the hands of the people who love them. A spouse's trembling goodbye before anesthesia. A parent squeezing a child's hand. A nervous teenager staring at the ceiling while rolling into the OR. These moments settle quietly into your memory.

Some cases follow you home. Trauma cases. Pediatric cases. Cancer resections. Emergency C-sections where two lives hang in balance. Cases where the room shifts from routine to life-or-death in seconds. Your hands stay steady, but your heart remembers.

And then there are the victories — the operations where a tumor is removed cleanly, where a broken bone is restored, where a transplant finds its home, where a patient's life restarts. You feel those wins too.

Over time, you learn emotional boundaries. You protect your heart enough to function, but not so much that you lose empathy. You let emotion inform your humanity, not disrupt your performance.

Some techs journal. Some debrief with coworkers. Some find closure through rituals — a quiet moment at the scrub sink, a deep breath before leaving the OR, a shared word with the team.

Emotional attachment doesn't make you weak.

It makes you human.

And humanity has a place in the OR — even behind the mask.

Q20. How do you recover after a difficult case?

Recovery begins the moment the case ends, even if you don't realize it. Your body comes down from the adrenaline. Your hands may shake. Your breathing may deepen. Your brain replays the moment when everything changed — the complication, the bleeding, the urgency, the things you had to do without hesitation.

The first step is **acknowledgment**. Difficult cases take a toll. Surgical Technologists often shoulder responsibility quietly — the sterility they protected, the instruments they prepared, the speed they maintained. You don't dismiss that weight. You honor it.

Next comes **debriefing**. Sometimes formally, sometimes informally. You talk with your team:

"What went well?"

"What didn't?"

"What will we do differently next time?"

These discussions aren't blame sessions — they're growth sessions. They transform fear into skill.

Then, there's **physical reset**. Water. Food. A few minutes in the break room. A long walk to the elevator and back. Stretching your hands after holding retractors for hours. The OR demands endurance; recovery restores it.

Emotionally, you find your own rhythm. Some techs sit quietly in their car before driving home. Some lean on coworkers who understand the unspoken language of OR hardship. Some release emotion through tears, while others feel numb for a while. All of it is normal.

Reflection comes later — in the shower, on the couch, lying in bed. You think about the patient. You think about your role. You think about what you learned.

And then a powerful truth emerges:

You did your job.

You stood in the storm and stayed steady.

You showed up in the moment that mattered most.

Recovery is not forgetting the case.

It's honoring your strength and preparing for the next one.

Q21. How do Surgical Technologists handle long surgeries that last 6, 8, or even 12 hours?

Long surgeries test your endurance, focus, emotional stamina, hydration, and physical conditioning. They require a different level of preparation — and a different level of mental discipline.

First, your setup must be flawless. In a long case, you won't have the luxury of stepping away for supplies or rethinking your layout. Everything must be accessible, organized, and intuitive so that even hours into the case, your muscle memory can guide your hands.

Hydration and nutrition matter. Experienced techs drink water before scrubbing in and pack protein bars to eat between turnovers. Once you scrub in, you're committed — no food, no bathroom, no breaks unless your relief arrives.

Body mechanics are essential. Techs shift weight, adjust foot placement, micro-bend knees, reposition retractors, and occasionally rotate their shoulders to prevent fatigue. Standing rigid is the enemy. Subtle, constant adjustments keep your body from breaking down.

Your mind enters a different mode during long cases. You learn how to maintain hyper-focus during critical moments, then soften your awareness during slower parts while staying vigilant. You protect your mental energy the way athletes pace themselves during marathons.

Breaks, when available, are strategic. You eat quickly. Stretch intentionally. Reset your breath. Then return with renewed clarity.

Emotionally, the OR team becomes your anchor. The surgeon's pacing, the anesthesiologist's calm, the nurse's rhythm — they sustain you. You lean on each other quietly.

Long surgeries aren't endurance tests you suffer through.

They are acts of sustained professionalism, presence, and discipline that prove you belong in the OR.

Q22. What makes a Surgical Technologist truly exceptional?

Exceptional Surgical Technologists aren't defined by speed or memorization — though both matter. They stand out because they elevate the entire OR with their presence, mindset, and mastery.

First, they anticipate with intuition, not guesswork. They understand not just the steps but the *story* of the procedure — when tension rises, when complications are likely, when to move closer, when to back off.

Second, exceptional techs know their instruments deeply. They catch defects others miss. They organize trays with strategic elegance. Their Mayo stand is clean, logical, and effortless to navigate.

Third, they protect the sterile field with near-religious devotion. They see contamination before it happens. They prevent it without drama. They understand sterility as a living discipline, not a rulebook.

Fourth, they stay emotionally steady. Exceptional techs do not escalate tension — they absorb it. Their calm becomes the room's calm.

Fifth, they communicate with clarity. They don't shout. They don't freeze. They speak with professionalism and presence:

"Knife down."

“Heavy forceps coming your way.”

“Count correct.”

Their communication makes the room safer.

Sixth, they learn constantly. They study preference cards. They ask senior techs for advice. They stay curious, humble, and hungry.

Finally, they care — quietly but deeply. They know the patient will never see their face, but they treat every step like someone’s life depends on it.

Because it does.

Exceptional techs don’t just do the job.

They define the standard.

Q23. How important is teamwork in the OR for Surgical Technologists?

Teamwork is not an optional skill in the OR — it is the foundation of safety, efficiency, and survival in a high-stakes environment. Surgery is never a solo act. It is a choreography of roles: the surgeon, the anesthesiologist, the circulating nurse, and the Surgical Technologist.

For techs, teamwork begins before the patient arrives. You coordinate with the circulator on equipment needs, room setup, table configuration, and patient positioning. You communicate openly about potential issues: missing instruments, outdated preference cards, malfunctioning equipment. Silence is not safety — communication is.

During the case, teamwork becomes synchronization. The surgeon relies on your anticipation and precision. The circulator relies on your sterile awareness. Anesthesia relies on your stability during positioning and transitions. Even the smallest gesture — a glance, a nod, a hand movement — can communicate volumes.

Teamwork also means humility. You accept help. You give help. You know when to step forward and when to step back. You never let ego threaten safety.

And when things go wrong — because in the OR, they sometimes do — teamwork becomes your greatest defense. The surgeon may tighten their voice. Anesthesia may call out concerns. The nurse may scramble for supplies. Your calm presence and coordinated response help stabilize the entire room.

At the end of the day, the OR works because the people inside it work together.

Teamwork isn't just important — it's everything.

Q24. What is the role of Surgical Technologists in preventing surgical site infections (SSI)?

Preventing surgical site infections is one of the most critical responsibilities of Surgical Technologists. You are the primary guardian of sterility — the gatekeeper between the patient's vulnerable tissues and the outside world.

Your role begins with **proper sterile technique**. Every single action — from opening supplies to moving around the table — is either protecting or endangering the sterile field. You maintain strict awareness of boundaries. You don't reach over nonsterile areas. You don't allow clutter or confusion on your Mayo stand.

You ensure all instruments are sterile, intact, and functioning. You inspect trays for biological indicators, moisture, tears, cracks, or packaging compromise. You reject anything that isn't perfect.

You control contamination risks throughout the case. If a glove tears, you change it. If a drape shifts, you adjust it. If someone brushes too close, you call it out. You do this without hesitation, because the risk of silence is too great.

You also reduce infection risk through efficiency. The faster and smoother the case flows, the less time the wound remains open. Your anticipation shortens operative time and improves safety.

At closure, your counts, irrigations, and handling of dressings further protect the patient.

A Surgical Technologist doesn't just *follow* sterile technique.

You embody it.

You enforce it.

You protect it as if someone's life depends on it —

because it does.

Q25. How do Surgical Technologists handle mistakes?

Mistakes in the OR feel heavier than mistakes anywhere else — because the stakes are higher. But every Surgical Technologist learns the same truth: mistakes happen. What defines your professionalism is how you respond.

First, you acknowledge the error immediately. If a glove tears, a contaminated item touches the field, or an instrument falls outside the sterile boundary, you speak up. Silence is unsafe. Honesty is protection.

Next, you correct it quickly. Change gloves. Replace instruments. Rebuild the field if necessary. You act decisively — not defensively — because your priority is always the patient.

Emotionally, mistakes sting. You replay them in your mind. You feel embarrassment, fear, or regret. But this processing is part of your growth, not your downfall. Every expert in the OR has made mistakes — but the best ones learned, adjusted, and never repeated them.

After the case, you reflect. What led to the mistake? Distraction? Fatigue? Inexperience? Poor positioning? Once you identify the cause, you develop a strategy to prevent it next time.

Mistakes don't make you a bad Surgical Technologist.

They make you a better one —

if you face them with honesty, humility, and a commitment to excellence.

Q26. What should a new Surgical Technologist expect during their first 90 days on the job?

Your first 90 days as a Surgical Technologist are an initiation — the moment you stop being a student studying surgery and start becoming someone who *lives* it. Expect to feel overwhelmed at first. The OR is its own ecosystem with its own culture, language, unspoken rules, and choreography.

You're suddenly surrounded by seasoned techs who move with a confidence you can't yet imagine having. That's normal.

Early on, you'll focus on mastering foundations: pulling cases correctly, organizing your back table, protecting the sterile field with instinctive awareness, performing counts with confidence, and learning surgeon preferences. You won't be perfect — and no one expects you to be — but they *will* expect effort, humility, and a willingness to learn.

During this period, you'll shadow experienced techs who scrub the most complex cases. Pay attention to their hands, their timing, the way they speak, and the rhythm they create. These details will become part of your operating style.

Emotionally, the first 90 days teach resilience. Some days you'll feel proud; other days you'll feel like you know nothing at all. That's part of the curve. What matters is how you respond: take notes, ask questions, seek feedback, show up early, and prepare thoroughly.

The defining shift happens around week eight or nine:

You stop surviving.

You start *adapting*.

You begin anticipating small steps, catching potential issues, and feeling moments of confidence.

By Day 90, you may not feel like an expert (you're not supposed to), but you'll feel something new: belonging.

Q27. How do Surgical Technologists collaborate with circulating nurses?

The Surgical Technologist and the circulating nurse are the backbone of the OR — two different roles, one shared mission. Collaboration between the two is essential for flow, safety, and patient outcomes.

Before the case, you review preference cards together, discuss positioning needs, clarify supplies, and anticipate challenges. The circulator retrieves equipment from outside the sterile field while you prepare and protect the sterile environment itself. You are the hands inside the field; they are the hands everywhere else.

During surgery, communication becomes a quiet dialogue. The circulator listens for your verbal cues:

“Knife down.”

“Suture coming back.”

“Need another suction tip.”

They manage supply flow, secure specimens, monitor the room, chart events, assist anesthesia, and anticipate needs based on what they see happening at your field.

You, in turn, rely on the circulator to keep the room moving smoothly. A good circulator senses your tempo, recognizes when tension rises, and supports you before you even ask. You respect each other’s roles — you don’t reach outside your boundary, and they don’t cross into yours without a purpose.

After the case, the teamwork continues as you perform counts together, verify instrument returns, and reset the room for the next patient.

The most successful ST–circulator teams communicate clearly, trust deeply, and support each other consistently. When that partnership clicks, the OR becomes unstoppable.

Q28. How do Surgical Technologists manage multiple surgeons with different preferences?

Every surgeon is their own universe. They have distinct styles, rhythms, temperaments, and quirks. One may want silence; another may talk nonstop. One may hold instruments delicately; another may move with force and speed. Your job is not to standardize them — it's to synchronize with them.

You begin with preference cards, but you quickly learn they are snapshots, not whole stories. Real preferences reveal themselves in the room. One surgeon may love a specific retractor that isn't listed. Another may switch suture brands mid-procedure. One may want instruments passed horizontally instead of vertically.

The key is observation. You watch their hands, listen to their tone, notice their pacing. You store these details mentally — or in a notebook if allowed. You don't rely solely on memory until experience makes it second nature.

Adaptability is essential. In a single day, you might work with a surgeon who jokes through cases followed immediately by one who barely speaks. You change your communication style accordingly. The best STs speak every surgeon's "language."

Anticipation also shifts from surgeon to surgeon. If Dr. A always uses suction early, you prep it ahead of schedule. If Dr. B prefers a specific clamp during dissection, you keep it close. If Dr. C gets frustrated by delays, you pre-open sutures or instruments strategically.

Managing multiple surgeons isn't stressful once you accept one truth:

Preferences aren't obstacles — they're invitations to expertise.

Learning them elevates you from being a good tech to being an exceptional one.

Q29. How does a Surgical Technologist support surgeries involving robotics?

Robotic surgery transforms the Surgical Technologist into a hybrid role — part scrub tech, part robotics technician, part systems specialist. Your responsibilities begin long before the incision.

First, you ensure the robotic system is inspected, cleaned, and functioning. You gather the proper robotic instruments, inspect their tips and joints, verify expiration dates, load cartridges, and prepare the sterile drapes designed specifically for the robot's arms.

During setup, you help position the robot relative to the patient — precise angles, distances, and docking points matter. Once anesthesia completes positioning, you coordinate with the team to dock each robotic arm at the correct port.

When the surgeon moves to the console, *you* become the hands at the bedside. You load instruments into robotic arms, change them when they wear down or get contaminated, troubleshoot robotic error messages, and adjust the arms if they collide or drift.

In robotic surgery, timing is everything. If the surgeon needs an instrument replaced, they rely entirely on your speed and accuracy. The smoother your hands, the smoother the entire case.

Robotic surgery also requires a deeper understanding of anatomy, because you're often assisting in very tight spaces with magnified, high-definition visuals. You learn how robotic needles differ from traditional ones, how articulating tips behave, and how to maintain instrument integrity.

You are not simply supporting the robot —

you are the bridge between human precision and robotic capability.

That makes your role both highly specialized and increasingly valuable in the future OR.

Q30. What should students know before entering a Surgical Technology program?

Students often imagine the OR through TV shows — glamorous, dramatic, adrenaline-filled moments. And while the OR is incredible, students should enter their program with grounded expectations and open minds.

First, the academics are rigorous. Anatomy, microbiology, surgical procedures, sterile technique, instrument identification — these aren't memorized casually. They require repetition, discipline, and focused studying. The people who thrive are the ones who treat it like a profession from day one.

Second, clinicals will stretch you. You will stand for hours, feel lost, struggle to identify instruments under pressure, and occasionally feel like an imposter. That's part of the process. Growth happens in the discomfort.

Third, communication skills are essential. You'll learn how to speak concisely, professionally, and respectfully — especially when tensions run high. You'll learn OR etiquette: who you talk to, when you talk, and how tone shapes the room.

Fourth, you must develop thick skin. Surgeons may speak abruptly. Nurses may correct you. Techs may push you to improve. None of it is personal. It is all part of preparing you for a space where mistakes matter.

Fifth, curiosity is your greatest asset. Ask questions. Watch everything. Lean into repetition — it's how you build confidence.

Finally, students should know this: Surgical Technology is a calling. It demands resilience, precision, humility, and a strong sense of purpose. But if you commit to the journey, it becomes one of the most rewarding careers in healthcare.

Q31. How important is speed for a Surgical Technologist?

Speed matters in the OR — but never more than accuracy, safety, and anticipation. Fast hands mean nothing if they deliver the wrong instrument. Rapid movement means nothing if it disrupts sterility. The goal isn't to be the fastest tech — it's to be the smoothest.

In your early months, speed will feel elusive. Every movement seems to take too long because you're thinking through every step. But with practice, muscle memory develops. You begin setting up trays faster. You pass instruments more confidently. You transition between steps with fluidity.

Speed becomes a natural byproduct of competence.

But here's the nuance: The OR values *controlled* speed. The kind of speed that feels calm, intentional, and unhurried even when you're moving quickly. The kind that lowers risk rather than raising it. The kind that creates flow instead of chaos.

True speed is quiet. It looks like:

- A tech who has every instrument perfectly placed before the surgeon arrives.

- A tech who anticipates three steps ahead so there's no delay in the sequence.

- A tech who never searches — because everything is exactly where it belongs.

- A tech who prevents problems before they happen, which saves time more than any fast hand ever could.

Surgeons don't praise "speedy" techs —

they praise techs who make cases feel effortless.

Q32. What is the emotional toll of working in surgery day after day?

The emotional toll of Surgical Technology is real — it accumulates quietly, behind the mask, behind the sterile field, behind the focus you bring to every case. You witness life-changing moments without ever being part of the patient's story. You carry stress the patient never sees and responsibility the public rarely understands.

There are cases that leave marks on you. Pediatric emergencies. Traumas where outcomes shift suddenly. Cancer resections where the weight of the diagnosis hangs over the room. Obstetric emergencies where two lives depend on seconds.

You are trained to stay composed, but you're still human. You may cry in your car after work. You may feel numb. You may dream about the cases that shook you. You may feel the quiet ache of carrying emotions you never voiced aloud.

There's also the emotional fatigue of OR culture — the intensity, the personalities, the demand for perfection. The expectation that you'll function under pressure day after day.

But there is also emotional reward. Cases that save lives. Moments of teamwork that feel transcendent. Days where everything goes exactly right and you feel proud, grounded, and essential.

Healthy techs learn emotional hygiene: talking to peers, debriefing after tough cases, maintaining hobbies outside healthcare, resting deeply, and understanding that it is okay to feel.

You don't have to be unbreakable to belong in the OR.

You only have to be willing to keep showing up — and to seek support when the job becomes heavy.

Q33. How does a Surgical Technologist build trust with surgeons?

Trust isn't built in a single case — it's built in a thousand small moments. And surgeons, who rely on precision and predictability, develop trust based on consistency, not personality.

First, you show up prepared. When a surgeon enters and sees their instruments perfectly laid out, sutures organized, and trays checked, they notice. Preparation builds credibility before you ever pass the first instrument.

Next, you demonstrate anticipation. When you hand the surgeon what they need before they ask — even once — it shifts their perception of you. Repeat it consistently, and trust grows.

You also communicate with purpose. Short, clear phrases. No unnecessary noise. No defensiveness. You speak in a way that supports the flow of the room.

Protecting the sterile field consistently builds immense trust. Surgeons feel unsafe when sterility is questionable. When you enforce standards calmly and confidently, they trust you with the most important safety layer of the case.

Finally, trust grows when you stay calm — especially when things go wrong. A tech whose hands remain steady under pressure is priceless to a surgeon.

Over time, surgeons stop explaining every step. They start relying on your rhythm. They start requesting you by name.

Trust is earned.

And once you earn it, you become part of their surgical identity.

Q34. What role does intuition play in Surgical Technology?

Intuition in the OR is not mystical — it's the result of

disciplined observation, repetition, and pattern recognition. But once developed, it feels like a sixth sense.

Techs with strong intuition can feel the shift in the room before anyone speaks. They know when a surgeon is about to ask for suction based on the angle of their shoulders. They sense when a tension suture is coming based on how tissue behaves. They predict complications because they've seen the early signs before: a sudden change in lighting, a quiet shift in anesthesia, a subtle urgency in the surgeon's hands.

Intuition tells you when to open additional supplies, when to move closer to the field, when to prepare backup instruments, and when to stay still. It guides your timing — the difference between interrupting a surgeon's flow and supporting it seamlessly.

Developing intuition takes time. At first, everything feels conscious: "What comes next? What do I hand?" But as experience accumulates, your subconscious begins running parallel with the case, tracking patterns and expectations.

Intuition makes you faster, safer, and more reliable. It transforms you from a technician into a partner.

In the OR, intuition is not an accessory —

it's an essential tool in the tech's toolkit.

Q35. How do Surgical Technologists prevent burnout?

Burnout creeps into the OR through fatigue, emotional strain, understaffing, overtime, tense cases, and unrelenting precision. Preventing burnout requires proactive care — not just hope.

Techs protect themselves by developing healthy boundaries. They take breaks when available, stretch during turnovers, hydrate, and avoid carrying emotional weight home without processing it.

Rotating through specialties helps too. Spending weeks only in trauma or ortho can drain even the strongest tech. Variety keeps your mind stimulated and your emotions balanced.

Healthy techs also speak up — not aggressively, but assertively. They request relief during long cases. They ask for help lifting heavy trays. They advocate for safe staffing ratios. Silence accelerates burnout; communication slows it.

Social support is essential. OR teams often become families, and techs rely on coworkers who understand the unique pressures of the job. These relationships protect mental well-being more than any policy ever could.

Off the job, self-care is nonnegotiable. Sleep, exercise, hobbies, and non-medical friends help restore a sense of identity beyond scrubs and sterile fields.

Most importantly, techs prevent burnout by remembering their why. The OR is intense, but it is also meaningful. Reconnecting with purpose — with the lives you help change — brings resilience.

You can't pour endlessly from an empty cup.

Preventing burnout means learning to refill it intentionally.

Q36. What's the difference between a good ST and a great one?

Good Surgical Technologists know the steps. Great ones know the story.

A good tech follows the sequence, performs counts accurately, sets up trays well, and passes instruments correctly. They are functional, dependable, and safe.

A great tech is something more.

Great techs anticipate without being asked. They sense the surgeon's rhythm and adjust instinctively. They prep instruments the surgeon didn't know they needed yet. They prepare contingency plans quietly — a backup clamp, a different retractor, an extra suture.

Great techs maintain calm energy in the room. They don't feed tension; they dissolve it. They move with intention, never rushing, never panicking. Their presence stabilizes the team.

Great techs know instruments deeply — how they behave, how they break, how they're repaired, and when they should be replaced. Their Mayo stands look like art: clean, intuitive, efficient.

Great techs communicate professionally. They don't make excuses. They don't escalate conflict. They bring clarity and confidence.

Great techs mentor new students with patience. They lift others rather than gatekeeping knowledge.

Great techs are trusted — not requested occasionally, but demanded by surgeons because they elevate the entire case.

The difference is simple:

A good tech supports the operation.

A great tech *defines* it.

Q37. Are Surgical Technologists involved in patient positioning?

Yes — Surgical Technologists play a critical role in patient positioning, even though the circulating nurse and anesthesia provider have primary responsibility. Positioning is a multi-person, safety-critical process, and you are an essential part of the team.

Before positioning begins, you review the surgeon's preference card and procedure notes to determine the required position: supine, lithotomy, prone, lateral, or modified variations. Each position has its own risks and requires specific padding, stabilization, and support equipment.

You help gather supplies — stirrups, gel pads, arm boards, safety straps, axillary rolls, blankets — and ensure they're available before anesthesia induces the patient.

During positioning, you support the patient's limbs, help secure the arms, assist with lifts or rolls, and confirm that bony prominences are padded. You must be gentle, precise, and communicative. The patient is unconscious and vulnerable; your care prevents nerve injuries, pressure injuries, and postoperative complications.

After positioning, you help apply skin prep, drapes, and equipment such as the robot or imaging systems. You double-check that no wires, tubes, or lines are kinked or compressed.

Positioning is more than logistics —

it is an act of protecting a patient who cannot protect themselves.

And that makes the ST's role essential.

Q38. What does the "sterile conscience" mean in Surgical Technology?

A "sterile conscience" is the ethical foundation of Surgical Technology. It means that you uphold sterile technique even when no one is watching — even when it's inconvenient, uncomfortable, or unpopular. It is your internal standard, your commitment to the patient, and your willingness to speak up the moment contamination occurs.

A sterile conscience means you don't rationalize breaches. If your glove touches a nonsterile surface, you change it. If a drape shifts, you fix it. If an instrument falls outside the field, you replace it. You do not hope no one noticed — you act because you know the patient's safety depends on you.

It also means you hold others accountable respectfully. If a surgeon reaches too far, if a circulator leans close to the field, if a student makes an error, you speak up. Not with shame — with clarity and professionalism.

A sterile conscience requires humility. It admits mistakes quickly because hesitation risks harm. It recognizes your humanity and the gravity of your responsibility.

The strongest Surgical Technologists are not the fastest or the most experienced.

They are the ones with uncompromising sterile conscience —

because they never let convenience outweigh safety.

Q39. How do Surgical Technologists support laparoscopic procedures?

Laparoscopic surgery transforms the OR into a video-guided universe, and Surgical Technologists play a key technical and procedural role.

Before the case, you gather specialized equipment: trocars, insufflation tubing, laparoscopic graspers, scissors, dissectors, clip appliers, and energy devices. You ensure the laparoscope is clean, the camera works, and the light cord is functioning.

You also prepare insufflation equipment — CO_2 flow, pressure settings, and tubing connections — because without proper insufflation, the surgeon cannot visualize the operative field.

During the case, you pass laparoscopic instruments through trocars, load clip appliers, manage sutures, and help navigate the patient's anatomy through screens. Laparoscopic cases require heightened awareness because instruments are long, angles are awkward, and visual cues replace tactile ones.

You manage fogging, clean the lens frequently, adjust camera angles, and anticipate when the surgeon needs suction, irrigation, or energy.

Your ability to maintain clear visualization directly affects safety and speed.

Laparoscopy is a dance between technology and touch —

and the Surgical Technologist is the one who keeps that dance moving.

Q40. How does a Surgical Technologist handle personality conflicts within the OR team?

The OR is full of strong personalities — surgeons with high expectations, nurses balancing multiple demands, anesthesia providers managing critical physiology, and techs who often carry the emotional weight of the field. Conflict is inevitable, but how you handle it defines your professionalism.

First, you stay neutral. You don't engage in gossip, alliances, or drama. You remain focused on patient safety and room flow. This neutrality earns respect.

Second, you communicate with clarity and calmness. "What do you need?" "Let's reset." "How can we fix this quickly?" These phrases de-escalate conflict and keep the room functional.

Third, you avoid reacting emotionally. Tone may rise. Criticism may occur. Pressure may intensify. You respond with measured professionalism instead of matching intensity.

Fourth, you set quiet boundaries. If a surgeon repeatedly uses disrespectful language, you can speak privately with a charge nurse. If a coworker undermines your work, you address it off the sterile field with honesty and respect.

Finally, you focus on the patient. In the OR, there is always one truth that dissolves most conflicts:

The person on the table matters more than anyone's ego.

When you hold to that truth, you become a grounding force — and conflict loses its power.

Q41. How do Surgical Technologists support orthopedic surgeries involving implants and hardware?

Orthopedic surgery transforms a Surgical Technologist into part mechanic, part engineer, and part procedural strategist. These cases revolve around hardware — plates, screws, rods, nails, trials, guides, jigs, and power tools — and the tech is the person who orchestrates every piece so the surgeon can reconstruct bone with precision.

Prep begins long before the patient enters the room. You inspect trays containing dozens of specialized instruments, some with moving parts that must be tested for function. Orthopedic trays are heavy, stacked, and often intimidating at first glance. Over time, you learn the anatomy of each one: where the depth gauges live, which screwdrivers match which screw sets, how to assemble guides, and how to troubleshoot power equipment that refuses to cooperate.

During the case, your anticipation becomes as important as your hands. Ortho surgeons often move quickly, relying on you to have the next drill bit, plate, or reduction clamp ready before they ask. You learn the rhythm of fracture reduction, the sequence of joint replacement, and the muscle memory of passing tools that are heavier and more complex than in other specialties.

Implants require impeccable organization. You manage the implant rep, verify sizes, open sterile implants without contamination, and track every screw and component used. Documentation must be perfect — implants follow patients for life.

You also monitor sterility constantly. Orthopedic cases involve movement, repositioning, large fields, and bulky equipment. Maintaining clean boundaries is a full-time job.

Supporting orthopedic surgeries isn't just about tools — it's about precision, timing, and the ability to turn mechanical reconstruction into smooth surgical choreography.

Q42. How do Surgical Technologists work alongside surgical residents and fellows?

Residents and fellows bring a unique energy to the OR — a mix of eagerness, intensity, curiosity, and sometimes nervousness as they learn their craft. For Surgical Technologists, working with them is part mentorship, part collaboration, and part safeguarding the flow of the room.

Residents rely on you more than they'll ever admit. They look to you for the right instruments, for cues about sterile field management, and for subtle guidance on surgical sequence. You often become the quiet teacher:

"This retractor works better for exposure here."

"Keep your hand positioned like this."

"Watch the drape — you're close to breaking sterility."

You support without overstepping. You guide without condescension. You help them succeed because their success is tied to patient safety.

At the same time, residents may deviate from the attending surgeon's usual preferences, and you must adapt quickly. One resident may want long instruments; another may prefer short. One may take extra time during dissection; another may move too fast. You learn to read each personality and adjust your style accordingly.

Fellows — having already completed residency — often carry advanced skill but still appreciate your expertise with instruments and room flow. Many fellows treat techs as essential surgical partners.

Your greatest contribution to residents and fellows is stability. They are learning. They make mistakes. They get corrected. They feel pressure. Your calm presence helps anchor the room.

Surgical Technologists don't just support operations –

they support the people becoming surgeons.

Q43. What challenges do Surgical Technologists face when working in trauma centers?

Trauma centers redefine everything you think you know about surgical rhythm. Cases don't wait. They burst into the OR with speed, unpredictability, and emotion. The biggest challenges for techs in trauma settings revolve around pace, readiness, variability, and emotional load.

The first challenge is **volume and unpredictability**. You may be in the middle of a routine procedure when trauma paging begins. Suddenly, two additional rooms open, and you must help set up quickly, pull trays, and think three steps ahead while adrenaline fills the air.

Second, trauma cases don't follow standard sequences. You may prepare for an exploratory laparotomy only to shift the focus to vascular control or rapid packing. Adaptability becomes your superpower.

Third, instrumentation varies widely. Trauma touches every specialty: orthopedic fractures, abdominal bleeding, thoracic wounds, neurosurgical emergencies. You must know a bit of everything – and know how to pivot fast.

Fourth, trauma cases often require complex teamwork. Anesthesia may struggle to stabilize the patient. Nurses may be juggling multiple rooms. Surgeons may move with urgency you haven't seen before. You remain calm to counterbalance the chaos.

Finally, trauma techs absorb emotional weight. Some cases end well. Some don't. Some stay in your memory forever. Recovery involves processing, leaning on coworkers, and learning not to carry every case home.

Trauma is demanding, but it is also one of the most meaningful environments for growth. It tests you, teaches you, and reveals your strength.

Q44. How do Surgical Technologists support neurosurgery cases with delicate instrumentation?

Neurosurgery feels like stepping into a sacred, quieter version of the OR. Everything is slower, softer, and more deliberate. Surgical Technologists support these cases by mastering micro-instruments, precision sequencing, and the calm energy that defines neurosurgical work.

Before the case, you inspect instruments with extraordinary attention to detail. Neurosurgical tools are delicate, slender, and highly specialized — from micro scissors and fine forceps to bipolar cautery tips the size of eyelash hairs. A bent tine or dulled edge can compromise the entire procedure.

You prepare specialized trays such as craniotomy sets, spinal sets, microdissection sets, and neuronavigation equipment. Neurosurgery also often requires advanced technology like stereotactic systems, microscopes, and drills with ultra-fine burrs. You ensure everything is functional before draping begins.

During surgery, your instrument passing becomes quieter and more controlled. Sudden motions disrupt the surgeon's concentration. You handle instruments as if they are extensions of the surgeon's fingers — because they are. Anticipation becomes art: knowing when to offer suction gently, when to present microdebridement tools, when to adjust the microscope view.

Because neurosurgery often involves long cases in stillness, you must maintain stamina while staying mentally engaged.

Supporting neurosurgery isn't just technical —

it requires presence, respect, and the steadiness of a person who understands the gravity of where the surgeon's hands are.

Q45. How do Surgical Technologists manage specimen handling during surgery?

Specimen handling is one of the most legally and medically significant responsibilities in the OR. Every tissue sample, biopsy, culture, or foreign object must be handled with precision, labeled correctly, and delivered safely — because the diagnosis hinges on it.

As a Surgical Technologist, you begin by communicating clearly with the circulator:

"What type of specimen is this?"

"Is it fresh, in formalin, or sent dry?"

"Is it for pathology, culture, or microbiology?"

You ensure the sterile field remains intact while preparing the specimen for transfer. If sutures or markers indicate margins, you confirm orientation with the surgeon. Mistakes here can alter cancer staging or surgical planning.

Timing matters. Some specimens must be sent immediately, while others await the end of the case. Cultures require sterile technique. Tumor samples may require special containers. Orthopedic hardware removed during revision surgery must be documented.

During transfer, sterility and accuracy are everything. You place the specimen in a sterile container, verify labeling, verbally confirm with the circulator, and then release it.

The responsibility is weighty:

A mislabeled specimen can lead to a misdiagnosis.

A contaminated specimen can invalidate results.

A lost specimen can alter the patient's entire treatment plan.

Handling specimens isn't just a task —

it's a safeguard for the patient's medical future.

Q46. What is it like working with traveling Surgical Technologists?

Traveling Surgical Technologists bring a unique blend of experience, independence, and adaptability into the OR. They've seen dozens of hospitals, hundreds of surgeons, and countless variations of the same procedures — and that makes them valuable team members who elevate the entire room.

Working with travelers exposes you to new techniques,

unfamiliar approaches, and creative instrument setups. They often bring solutions you've never considered:

"Try organizing your Mayo like this — it saves movement."

"This surgeon at my last hospital used this retractor differently; want to see?"

Travelers adapt fast. They can walk into a new OR, learn workflows quickly, and remain calm because they've already lived through unfamiliarity countless times.

But travelers also face challenges. Every hospital has different culture, equipment, and preference cards. As a staff tech, you become their guide: "This surgeon likes this suture," "This room has issues with the lights," "We store ortho trays over here."

The relationship becomes collaborative. You learn from their breadth; they learn from your depth.

When the team respects travelers, they become a tremendous asset — not only strengthening cases but raising the OR's collective skillset.

Q47. How do Surgical Technologists manage the emotional impact of pediatric surgery?

Pediatric surgery touches the heart in ways few other specialties do. Even though your focus must remain technical, the emotional gravity of seeing a child on an OR table remains profound.

Before the case, you prepare differently. Instruments are smaller. Supplies are specialized. Medication doses require extra attention. Everything must be perfect — because children's bodies respond differently to surgical stress.

When the child arrives, you see fear, innocence, and trust all wrapped into one. Parents linger at the door, hoping for miracles. You feel that weight, even as you focus on the sterile field.

During the case, the emotional stakes heighten. Children's anatomy is tiny, delicate, and unforgiving. Surgeons rely heavily on your precision. Mistakes are not tolerable. You become hyper-aware of instrument placement, counts, and sterility.

Emotionally, pediatric cases stay with you. The victories feel sweeter. The challenges feel heavier.

You learn coping mechanisms:

- Deep breaths before scrubbing in
- Debriefs after difficult cases
- Leaning on teammates who understand
- Journaling or private reflection

Pediatric surgery demands technical excellence and emotional maturity —

a combination that shapes you forever.

Q48. How do Surgical Technologists prepare for cardiac surgery?

Cardiac surgery requires a higher level of precision, readiness, and mental focus. These cases involve bypass machines, delicate instruments, and life-or-death decisions happening second to second. Preparation begins long before the patient enters the room.

You start by pulling highly specialized trays: sternal saw sets, vascular instrument sets, coronary artery bypass sets, graft handling tools, and micro suture assortments. You inspect every instrument — even minor defects can compromise the case.

You prepare equipment like warmers, cell savers, and hemostatic agents. You coordinate with perfusionists, who run the heart-lung machine. You familiarize yourself with graft materials, clamps, needle sizes, and sutures so thin they look like hair.

During the case, anticipation becomes everything. Cardiac surgeons rely on absolute precision. You pass instruments in a quiet, controlled manner. You protect the field with vigilance. You manage sutures carefully to avoid tangling. You prepare backup instruments before the surgeon asks.

Cardiac surgery demands your best self:

your sharpest mind, your calmest hands, your strongest sterile conscience.

Supporting cardiac surgery makes you a more disciplined, more confident, and more technically skilled Surgical Technologist.

Q49. How do Surgical Technologists learn the thousands of instrument names they must memorize?

Instrument memorization feels impossible at first — like learning a new language spoken only in metal. But over time, the OR teaches you through repetition, association, and pattern recognition.

You start with the basics: clamps, scissors, retractors, forceps. You learn shapes, sizes, and functions. Then you learn variations: curved vs. straight, toothed vs. smooth, long vs. short. You begin grouping instruments by family — all the Debakeys together, all the Kocher clamps, all the Army-Navys.

You practice by handling instruments daily. Muscle memory becomes your teacher. You quiz yourself during setup. You ask other techs questions — "Why does this surgeon prefer this?" "How is this different from that?"

The breakthrough moment comes when you stop memorizing and start understanding. You learn *why* an instrument exists. Why a surgeon chooses it. What tissue it's meant for. How it fits into the steps of the procedure.

Names follow function.

Function follows repetition.

Repetition builds mastery.

You don't learn instruments all at once —

you learn them one case, one tray, one day at a time.

Q50. What happens when a Surgical Technologist recognizes a potential complication before anyone else?

It happens more often than people think. Surgical Technologists, positioned at the sterile field, develop a view of the anatomy, instruments, and surgeon's hands that no one else in the room shares. Sometimes, your eyes catch things first: unexpected bleeding, tissue changes, unusual smells (burned tissue, infection), or equipment malfunction.

When you sense something, your first job is to stay calm. Panic disrupts the room. You communicate clearly, with respect and professionalism:

“Doctor, I’m noticing increased bleeding here.”

“This suction isn’t functioning; switching now.”

“This instrument seems compromised.”

Surgeons rely on your observations, especially during complex or fast-moving cases. They expect you to speak up promptly.

Your other job is to prepare. If you suspect vascular involvement, you bring vascular clamps closer. If bleeding increases, you set up additional suction or prepare sponges. If equipment fails, you reach for backups without hesitation.

Your intuition and vigilance can prevent complications from worsening —

and sometimes, they save lives.

Q51. How do Surgical Technologists handle long periods of silence in the OR?

Silence in the OR isn’t awkward — it’s sacred. It’s concentration, trust, rhythm. Long stretches of quiet often mean the surgeon is deep in the most delicate part of the case, and your job is to protect that stillness.

During silence, your awareness heightens. You monitor instrument placement, hand positioning, and field integrity. You pass items gently to avoid breaking focus. You watch for subtle cues — a shift in the surgeon's shoulders, a change in grip, a deep breath before a critical step.

Silence is where anticipation thrives. You sense the next step without words. You prepare instruments quietly. You open sutures slowly. You adjust lights or retractors with minimal motion.

Emotionally, silence can be grounding. It becomes a form of meditation — you're fully present, fully attuned, fully engaged.

Silence doesn't mean nothing is happening.

It means everything that matters is happening quietly.

Q52. How do Surgical Technologists adapt when a surgeon suddenly changes the surgical plan?

Surgical plans change for countless reasons: unexpected anatomy, complications, new findings, or a better approach. These moments test your adaptability, preparedness, and emotional control.

When a surgeon says, "We're switching to an open approach," "We need a different retractor," or "Prepare for vascular control," you respond with calm urgency. Panic has no place in this pivot.

You immediately pull the necessary trays or instruments, communicating with the circulator efficiently:

"We need the laparotomy set."

"Open vascular clamps."

"Bring additional suction."

You reorganize your field if needed. You protect sterility fiercely during sudden changes — the risk of contamination rises when the team moves quickly.

You anticipate sequence changes. If the surgeon shifts from laparoscopic to open, you prepare retractors, suction, sutures, and sponges appropriate for the new approach.

Adaptability is not improvisation —

it is preparation meeting reality.

The more specialties you master, the more confident you become when the plan changes.

And the OR respects a tech who handles pivots with stability.

Q53. How does a Surgical Technologist know when they're ready to specialize?

Specialization usually starts with a spark — a moment during a case when you feel unusually focused, unusually alive, or unusually connected to the work. Maybe it's the mechanical logic of orthopedics, the precision of neurosurgery, the adrenaline of trauma, or the calm complexity of robotics.

But timing matters. Most techs spend their first year gaining foundational skills before committing to a specialty. You know you're ready when:

- You feel confident in general surgery
- You manage counts without stress
- You anticipate routine steps easily
- You communicate clearly under pressure

- You troubleshoot problems independently
- Surgeons begin requesting you

Specializing is a natural evolution.

You're not leaving general surgery behind —

you're stepping into deeper mastery.

Q54. Why do so many Surgical Technologists love their job despite the pressure?

Because the OR is one of the few places where purpose is tangible. You see the immediate impact of your work. You see bones realigned, organs repaired, tumors removed, bleeding controlled, and lives saved. You witness transformation — and you help make it possible.

Techs love the adrenaline, the teamwork, the rhythm, the problem-solving, and the sense of belonging that comes from being part of a highly skilled, high-trust environment. They love learning new procedures, mastering instruments, and becoming experts in a world few people ever see closely.

They also love the identity the OR gives them.

A Surgical Technologist is someone who can stay calm under pressure, think quickly, work precisely, and protect patients in their most vulnerable moments.

Pressure doesn't define the job —

purpose does.

Q55. What advice do experienced Surgical Technologists give to new graduates?

The best advice from seasoned techs sounds simple but carries deep truth:

1. Be humble.

The OR will teach you more in one month than school did in a year.

2. Ask questions.

Curiosity prevents mistakes.

3. Watch experienced techs.

Their hands are libraries.

4. Prepare thoroughly.

Setup is half the battle.

5. Communicate professionally.

Your voice shapes the room.

6. Protect the sterile field above all else.

Safety is nonnegotiable.

7. Don't take tough feedback personally.

It's about the patient, not your ego.

8. Stay calm.

The room takes cues from your energy.

9. Learn instruments deeply.

Your confidence begins with mastery.

10. Take care of your body and mind.

This career is a marathon, not a sprint.

Experienced techs know the OR will challenge you —

but they also know it will shape you into someone stronger, steadier, and more capable than you imagined.

Q56. What should new Surgical Technologists know about working the night shift?

The night shift in the OR is a world of its own — quieter, darker, more intimate, and more unpredictable. New techs quickly learn that nighttime surgery isn't just "day shift at a different hour." It is a different rhythm, a different mindset, and sometimes a different version of yourself.

Nights usually run on smaller teams, which means everyone becomes more essential. You will often have one circulator, one anesthesia provider, and one tech covering multiple rooms. When trauma or emergencies hit, you feel the urgency at a deeper level because there aren't endless resources waiting down the hall.

Case variety skyrockets at night: ruptured appendixes, emergency C-sections, traumatic injuries, perforations, bleeds, and unexpected complications that couldn't wait until morning. You move from zero to full adrenaline in minutes.

The environment feels different too. Hallways are dim. Conversations are softer. There are no administrators, no visitors, fewer distractions. The work becomes about pure surgical focus — just you, the patient, and the team.

The biggest challenge is fatigue. You must learn how to pace yourself, hydrate, stretch, and maintain alertness during long, slow stretches followed by sudden bursts of intensity.

But nights also strengthen you more than any other shift. You learn autonomy, confidence, and calm under pressure. You discover that you're capable of far more than you knew. And you build a special bond with coworkers who share the quiet intensity of the night shift.

Working nights teaches resilience —

and resilience makes you a better Surgical Technologist in every environment.

Q57. What makes Surgical Technology a stable long-term career?

Surgical Technology remains one of the most stable careers in healthcare for several key reasons: consistently rising surgical volume, dependence on skilled OR teams, expanding surgical specialties, and the increasing complexity of procedures that require precision-oriented support.

First, surgeries aren't going away. As the population ages and chronic conditions increase, demand for surgical services grows. More surgeries means more techs. It's that simple.

Second, automation cannot replace Surgical Technologists. Robots may assist surgeons, but humans manage sterility, anticipate needs, troubleshoot equipment, and respond to unpredictable moments. The OR is too dynamic for full automation.

Third, specialty expansion creates career longevity. You can pivot into orthopedics, robotics, neurosurgery, cardiovascular procedures, ENT, ophthalmology, or trauma. If one area slows down, others remain strong.

Fourth, Surgical Technologists are central to OR efficiency. Hospitals rely on techs to maintain surgical flow, prevent errors, and reduce turnover time. Because the OR is one of the hospital's largest revenue centers, skilled techs are invaluable.

Job mobility also strengthens stability. You can work in hospitals, outpatient surgery centers, trauma centers, specialty clinics, labor and delivery units, and sterile processing leadership.

Finally, burnout can be mitigated through specialty changes, travel opportunities, shift variations, and career ladders such as certified first assistant roles or education.

Surgical Technology is not just stable —

it's future-proof.

Q58. How do Surgical Technologists support C-section deliveries in the OR?

C-sections blend surgical precision with the emotional intensity of childbirth. As a Surgical Technologist, your role is essential from setup to closure.

You begin by preparing the C-section tray, ensuring instruments for incision, retraction, clamping, suturing, and emergency interventions are ready. You also prepare supplies unique to obstetric surgery: cord clamps, uterine packs, suction bulbs, and neonatal equipment.

When the mother enters the OR, the energy shifts. There is anticipation, anxiety, and hope all at once. You maintain sterility while supporting a moment that is both medical and deeply human.

During the procedure, the pace changes rapidly. The initial incision is controlled and methodical. But once the uterus is opened, things move fast. The surgeon delivers the baby while you manage clamps, provide suction, prepare instruments for cord cutting, and hand tools with heightened speed.

The moment the baby cries — or doesn't — is unforgettable. The neonatal team takes over while the surgeons shift to repairing the uterus and abdominal layers.

Throughout the case, you maintain sterile technique, manage sutures, anticipate needs, and stay alert for complications like hemorrhage.

C-section cases are emotionally rich. They remind you that behind every incision is a family whose life changes in that moment.

Few surgical experiences feel as profound as helping bring a life safely into the world.

Q59. What does "anticipation" truly mean in the OR?

Anticipation is the invisible art that separates competent techs from extraordinary ones. It means understanding the procedure so thoroughly that you know what the surgeon needs before the surgeon knows they need it.

Anticipation begins with knowledge — memorizing procedural steps, identifying common variations, and studying each surgeon's personal style. But it evolves into intuition: noticing subtle cues, shifts in technique, and the small physical movements that reveal what's coming next.

A surgeon rotates their wrist slightly? They're switching from cutting to dissecting.

Their shoulders tense? Suction will be needed.

They pause for a beat? They're assessing anatomy for the next instrument.

You watch these cues like a language only you and the surgeon speak.

Anticipation also includes preparing for potential complications. If bleeding increases, you position clamps closer. If tissue thickens, you prepare longer instruments. You're always thinking two or three steps ahead.

The key to anticipation is not guesswork — it's preparation supported by deep understanding. You have the next instrument ready because you studied, you watched, you learned.

When anticipation is strong, the OR flows like a choreographed dance.

When it's weak, the OR stalls.

Anticipation makes you essential —

and surgeons remember techs who elevate their performance.

Q60. What should a Surgical Technologist do when a surgeon becomes frustrated or tense?

Surgeon frustration is part of OR life. It may stem from difficult anatomy, equipment issues, patient complexity, or external stressors. Your role is not to absorb the frustration — but to maintain stability in the room.

First, stay calm. Emotional reactions escalate tension; neutral energy diffuses it.

Second, continue passing instruments cleanly and confidently. Hesitation signals insecurity and can worsen the mood.

Third, troubleshoot quietly and effectively if equipment becomes an issue:

“This camera is fogging — swapping now.”

“Backup suction coming up.”

Clarity is your anchor.

Fourth, avoid taking comments personally. Surgeons use quick, blunt communication during high-pressure moments. It’s rarely about you.

Fifth, support the circulator. When the room becomes tense, teamwork becomes essential. You communicate cleanly, share a quick glance of understanding, and reinforce each other.

Finally, prioritize the patient above the atmosphere. Frustration is noise; the patient is the focus.

Your steady presence can reset the room.

A calm tech doesn’t just assist the surgery —

they safeguard the environment where healing happens.

Q61. How do Surgical Technologists handle sudden equipment failure?

Equipment failure is one of the most stressful OR moments — and one of the most defining tests of a Surgical Technologist’s composure. When something stops working, your job is to respond with speed, clarity, and precision.

First, you verbally identify the issue:

"The camera isn't receiving signal."

"The cautery is not cutting."

"The suction tubing is occluded."

This alerts the team immediately.

Second, you troubleshoot rapidly and systematically.

Is the cord loose?

Is the machine powered on?

Is the tip obstructed?

Is there a backup in the room?

Third, you communicate with the circulator:

"Please grab the backup camera head."

"We need the second suction setup."

"This cautery pencil isn't functioning — switching now."

You do not panic or apologize — you act.

Fourth, anticipate the surgeon's needs. If visualization is compromised, prepare sponges, lights, or additional suction. If cutting devices fail, prepare alternative tools.

Fifth, protect the sterile field even under pressure. Rushing increases contamination risk.

Finally, once stability returns, you mentally reset. Equipment failure shakes many new techs, but seasoned ones recognize it as part of OR life.

Technology fails.

People react.

Professionals respond.

Q62. How do Surgical Technologists handle multi-room coverage in a busy OR?

Multi-room coverage happens during high-volume days, emergencies, or when staffing is tight. It requires organization, efficiency, and the ability to prioritize under pressure.

You start by knowing your rooms — who's in which case, what phase each case is in, and what they'll need next. You mentally track time like a chess board.

When you float between rooms, communication is your anchor:

"What do you need before I step over to Room 7?"

"I'll be back in two minutes — calling for additional help now."

You prep instruments and supplies proactively. You assist in one room until the next critical step, then shift to the next room while keeping everyone informed.

You also lean on your team. Multi-room coverage works only when circulators, anesthesia, and techs communicate clearly and support each other without ego.

The biggest challenge is avoiding burnout. Multi-room days are mentally taxing. Pace yourself. Hydrate. Stretch. Breathe.

The OR rewards multitaskers —

but it respects those who maintain patient safety above all else.

Q63. How does stress affect Surgical Technologists, and how can they manage it effectively?

Stress in the OR is layered: technical, emotional, physical, and interpersonal. It accumulates in subtle ways — long cases, unexpected complications, surgeon conflicts, demanding schedules, and the intense responsibility of protecting the sterile field.

Recognizing stress symptoms is the first step: irritability, fatigue, difficulty concentrating, muscle tension, emotional detachment, or dread before shifts.

Effective management begins with boundaries. Take breaks. Stretch during turnovers. Hydrate. Remove yourself from the OR for a few minutes when possible.

Emotional processing is crucial. Debrief after difficult cases. Talk to teammates. Journal. Seek support if you're carrying too much alone.

Physical care matters too: sleep, nutrition, exercise, and rest days that truly disconnect you from the OR environment. Your body is your tool — replenish it.

Mindfulness and breathwork help significantly. Even a single slow inhale can reset your nervous system between intense moments.

Finally, perspective matters. Surgical Technologists are vital, skilled professionals — but they are still human. You will make mistakes, feel overwhelmed, and have tough days. That does not make you weak.

The OR demands strength —

but it also demands self-compassion.

Q64. How do Surgical Technologists maintain precision during extremely long surgeries?

Long surgeries — sometimes six, eight, or even twelve hours — require endurance, focus, and controlled energy. Maintaining precision over time is a skill.

Before the case, pacing is essential. You hydrate. You stretch. You mentally prepare. You know you're entering a marathon, not a sprint.

During the procedure, you use micro-breaks. When the surgeon pauses or shifts position, you gently flex your fingers, adjust your stance, roll your shoulders, or shift weight between feet. These small resets prevent fatigue from affecting performance.

Your setup matters too. Smart organization allows you to move less and think more. A well-designed Mayo stand reduces physical strain and improves efficiency.

Focus becomes rhythmic. You tune out distractions, stay anchored in the sequence, and maintain awareness of your hands and sterile field. If your mind wanders, you pull yourself back with intention.

Emotionally, you break the case into smaller mental segments. "Close part one," "Switching instruments," "Preparing sutures." This prevents the length from overwhelming you.

Long cases test everyone — but they also reveal your resilience.

Precision isn't just a skill; it's a disciplined mindset.

Q65. How do Surgical Technologists approach learning a new specialty?

Learning a new specialty is like learning a new surgical language. You begin by observing — watching experienced techs, studying instrument patterns, and listening for cues unique to the specialty.

You take notes. You memorize trays. You ask questions:

"What's the sequence here?"

"Why does the surgeon prefer this clamp?"

"How does this differ from general surgery?"

You also study anatomy specific to the specialty. Ortho requires bone knowledge; ENT requires familiarity with delicate head-and-neck structures; neuro requires understanding of cranial and spinal anatomy.

Hands-on practice accelerates learning. Setting up trays, practicing instrument assembly, and rehearsing steps builds confidence.

You accept that you'll feel lost at first — and that's normal. Mastery comes through repetition. Confidence comes from cumulative exposure.

Techs who embrace curiosity, humility, and persistence become specialists.

Specialists become indispensable.

Q66. How does the OR team respond when a Surgical Technologist catches a critical error?

When a tech catches a critical error — such as a count discrepancy, a sterility break, or a specimen issue — the OR team's reaction depends on the culture of the room, but professionally, it should always follow one principle:

If a tech speaks up, everyone listens.

Techs are guardians of the sterile field and instrument integrity. When you raise a concern, it signals potential risk to patient safety.

You might say:

"I'm missing a Ray-Tec on my count."

"This drape is contaminated."

"The specimen label does not match the patient."

The team pauses. The surgeon looks up. The circulator reassesses. The issue is addressed immediately.

In strong OR cultures, you are thanked for catching the error. In weaker cultures, you may encounter frustration — but patient safety still requires action.

Speaking up is never wrong. Silence is.

Your voice protects the patient —

and that is the OR's highest value.

Q67. How do Surgical Technologists handle high-turnover days with back-to-back cases?

High-turnover days feel like controlled chaos. You bounce from one case to the next with barely a moment to reset. Success requires planning, efficiency, and mental stamina.

Before the first case, you prepare multiple trays, sutures, and supplies for the entire day if possible. You review preference cards so you're not scrambling.

During turnovers, you work fast but never sacrifice setup quality. A sloppy setup leads to delays later — precision now saves time later.

You also communicate constantly with your circulator:

"I'll handle instruments; can you grab the implants?"

"I'll prep the Mayo while you confirm equipment."

When you anticipate steps well, you minimize delays.

Emotionally, you pace yourself. You breathe. You focus on one case at a time. High-turnover days test your endurance, not just your skills.

Techs who can thrive in high-turnover environments are invaluable —

and often requested by name.

Q68. What happens when a Surgical Technologist becomes the "go-to" person in the OR?

Becoming the "go-to" tech is a milestone. It means surgeons request you, nurses rely on you, and leadership trusts you to handle complex cases.

You're known for consistency, calmness, anticipation, and problem-solving. You elevate every room you enter.

But being the go-to tech also brings responsibility. You may receive more difficult cases, supervise students, help orient new staff, and troubleshoot equipment issues across rooms.

You become a resource — and a mentor.

You also gain leverage. When you speak, people listen. When you make suggestions about workflow, supplies, or safety, leadership pays attention.

Being the go-to tech is a badge of honor —

earned, never given.

Q69. Why do Surgical Technologists often feel a deep sense of pride in their work?

Because few careers place you so close to the heart of human healing. You witness transformation, precision, teamwork, and vulnerability. You see inside the human body — and inside moments where lives change.

Techs take pride in their mastery: the perfect setup, the flawless count, the seamless suture pass, the clean sterile field.

They also take pride in their resilience. Not everyone can handle the pressure, the blood, the hours, or the emotional intensity. The OR is a proving ground — and techs who thrive there feel pride because they've earned their place.

Most of all, pride comes from purpose.

Your hands help save lives.

Your vigilance prevents harm.

Your skill turns chaos into clarity.

You belong to a profession built on excellence —

and that pride stays with you.

Q70. What does growth look like for a Surgical Technologist over their first five years?

Growth in Surgical Technology is not linear — it's layered. Year one builds survival skills: sterile technique, instrument identification, room setup, communication basics, and emotional endurance.

Year two brings confidence. You anticipate steps, manage mid-level complexity, and begin syncing with surgeons.

Year three opens specialization opportunities. You gravitate toward orthopedics, neuro, robotics, or trauma. Surgeons begin to recognize your style.

Year four expands leadership. You precept students, train new hires, and take ownership of cases. You troubleshoot equipment, manage complex trays, and influence room flow.

Year five brings mastery. You feel at home in the OR. You maintain calm under pressure. You support complex cases with stability and precision. You are often requested by name.

Growth isn't just skill —

it's confidence, presence, and professional identity.

Q71. What role do Surgical Technologists play in preventing surgical site infections (SSIs)?

Preventing surgical site infections is one of the most important responsibilities of a Surgical Technologist — and it begins long before the first incision. SSIs are not random; they are prevented through disciplined sterile technique, environmental awareness, and constant vigilance.

Your first line of defense is preparation. You ensure instruments are properly sterilized, trays are intact, and all disposable items are opened without contamination. You organize your field efficiently so instruments remain clean and accessible.

During draping, your technique must be flawless. Drapes create the sterile field, and even a minor slip can introduce contamination. You guard the field like a shield — especially during movement or positioning.

Throughout the case, you watch everything: the surgeon's hands, the circulator's proximity, the edges of the drapes, the instrument tips, the count board, and your own sleeves and gloves. You speak up immediately if sterility is compromised, even if the room is tense. Silence is dangerous; action is protective.

Instrument management also matters. Instruments soiled with bioburden must be cleaned frequently. Items that hit below the table plane are considered contaminated. Sutures must remain dry and untouched by anything nonsterile.

You also help maintain environmental controls. Minimizing unnecessary traffic, ensuring proper gowning, and keeping movement deliberate all contribute to lower infection risk.

Finally, you model sterile conscience — the ethical commitment to protect the patient at all costs. SSIs can cause lifelong consequences. Your vigilance can prevent them entirely.

A Surgical Technologist does not merely assist in surgery —

they stand guard over the patient's safety.

Q72. How do Surgical Technologists collaborate with anesthesia providers?

Anesthesia providers — CRNAs and anesthesiologists — operate in a parallel universe to the surgeon. Their focus is physiology, hemodynamics, airway, and sedation. You, as the tech, work in harmony with them to create a seamless surgical experience.

Before the case, you ensure anesthesia has access to the head of the table, help secure the patient's arms and lines, and confirm that nothing in your setup obstructs monitors or equipment. Communication begins here:

"Is this positioning good for you?"

"Do you need access to this side?"

"Will we need additional padding or supports?"

During induction, you maintain situational awareness. You don't open sterile items too early. You avoid creating noise or motion that distracts anesthesia during airway management. If anesthesia requests a pause, you pause instantly.

Throughout the procedure, you monitor anesthesia's cues. If they ask for a quieter room, dim lights, additional suction, or time to stabilize the patient, you support them. You also help by managing cords and tubing to prevent tangles or accidental disconnections.

During emergence, you adjust your field to give anesthesia full access once again. You help with patient safety by securing instruments, stepping back appropriately, and preparing the room for transport.

Good anesthesia-tech collaboration keeps patients safe.

Great collaboration makes the entire OR feel like one mind working in synchrony.

Q73. How do Surgical Technologists contribute to surgical innovation and new technology adoption?

Surgical innovation doesn't succeed without Surgical Technologists — in fact, techs often determine whether new technology is adopted smoothly or not. When hospitals invest in robotics, advanced imaging systems, new staplers, or cutting-edge devices, it's the techs who learn the mechanics, troubleshoot issues, and teach others how to integrate them into workflow.

You become the bridge between vendors, surgeons, and the OR team. Vendors introduce the device, but you internalize it. You learn how it works, what breaks, what the backup plan is, and how to prep it quickly during high-stress cases. Surgeons rely on your knowledge; circulators rely on your familiarity; leadership relies on your feedback.

Innovation requires consistent setup, correct handling, and the ability to anticipate how technology alters the surgical flow. If a new power tool jams, you must know the reset sequence. If a novel implant has unique sizing, you must organize and track components. If a robot's arm needs recalibration, you must step in with confidence.

Techs also influence purchasing decisions. Your feedback on what works, what doesn't, and what slows turnover carries real weight. Leadership trusts the people using equipment daily.

In short, surgeons may pioneer new techniques —

but techs operationalize them.

Your expertise ensures innovation becomes not just possible, but practical.

Q74. How do Surgical Technologists handle emotionally difficult cases, such as loss of life?

Emotionally difficult cases are an unavoidable part of surgical life. Trauma patients who don't survive, emergency C-sections with devastating outcomes, complex cases where despite every effort the body cannot recover — these moments stay with you.

During the case, you remain composed because the team needs stability. You focus on technique, sterility, counts, and supporting the surgeon. But emotionally, you feel the weight, especially when the patient is young or the situation is unexpected.

When the case ends, the emotional impact often arrives in waves. Some techs step into the hallway to breathe. Some cry in private. Some need silence. Some debrief with coworkers who shared the moment. The OR is a family — and healing happens together.

Hospitals may offer formal debriefings or support systems, but many techs rely on each other. Talking about what you saw, what you felt, and what you feared helps release the emotional load.

Long-term, you develop resilience not by suppressing emotions, but by honoring them. You learn to compartmentalize without disconnecting. You build rituals: taking a walk after a hard case, journaling, listening to music, calling someone you trust.

You remind yourself that you did everything you could — and that the outcomes are not yours to carry alone.

Difficult cases shape you, soften you, and strengthen you.

They remind you why your presence in the OR matters.

Q75. What is the biggest misconception people have about Surgical Technologists?

The biggest misconception is that Surgical Technologists "just pass instruments." Nothing could be further from the truth.

People outside the OR rarely understand the depth of knowledge, technical skill, mental acuity, and emotional strength the role requires. Techs must memorize thousands of instruments, dozens of specialties, and hundreds of procedural sequences. They must understand anatomy, physiology, and surgical strategy well enough to anticipate needs before surgeons even verbalize them.

They maintain the sterile field — a responsibility with life-or-death implications. They manage equipment, troubleshoot technology, coordinate with anesthesia, protect patients from injury, and ensure the right instruments are used at the right time.

Techs also shoulder immense emotional labor. They support trauma cases, stillbirths, emergencies, and prolonged surgeries. They remain calm under pressure and carry internal resilience the public never sees.

Another misconception is that the job is static. In reality, techs grow continually — mastering new specialties, adapting to new technology, and evolving into leaders, educators, first assistants, and OR innovators.

Surgical Technologists are not instrument passers.

They are surgical partners — essential, skilled, and irreplaceable.

Q76. How do Surgical Technologists maintain efficiency without rushing?

Efficiency in the OR isn't speed — it's precision. Rushing causes contamination, mistakes, confusion, and tension. Efficiency means doing things correctly the first time, with smooth, intentional movements that conserve time and energy.

You begin with preparation: knowing the procedure, reviewing the preference card, understanding the surgeon's rhythm, and organizing your field intuitively. Thoughtful setup prevents frantic scrambling later.

During the case, efficiency comes from flow. You place instruments where your hands naturally move. You minimize unnecessary motions. You handle retractors with awareness, manage sutures cleanly, and keep the Mayo stand uncluttered.

You also communicate proactively.

"Suture ready."

"Next instrument on deck."

"Backup retractor available if needed."

This prevents delays without creating tension.

Efficiency is also mental. You stay present, focused, and attuned. You don't let fatigue or frustration interrupt your rhythm.

Ironically, the calmer you move, the faster the case feels —

because true efficiency is quiet, steady, and deliberate.

Q77. How do Surgical Technologists work with students shadowing in the OR?

Working with students is a privilege — and a responsibility. For many, observing you is their first glimpse into the OR. You are their introduction to sterile technique, surgical flow, professionalism, and the reality behind the mystique of surgery.

Your first job is to set expectations. You explain where they can stand, how to maintain sterility, what they can touch (usually nothing), and when they must speak softly or remain silent.

During the case, you narrate small insights when appropriate:

"This is the retractor we use to improve exposure."

"The surgeon prefers this suture for deeper layers."

"Watch how we maintain counts throughout."

You model professionalism, communication, and sterile conscience.

Students may ask questions that seem basic or awkward — remember, you were them once. Their curiosity is the spark that may lead them into this career.

You also protect the patient and the team. If a student gets too close to the sterile field, you correct them kindly but firmly. If they show anxiety, you guide them gently.

Mentorship is not about perfection. It's about presence.

Students remember techs who made them feel welcome —

and they model their future practice after those moments.

Q78. How do Surgical Technologists keep their skills sharp over time?

Skill maintenance requires intentional practice. Even experienced techs refresh their skills to stay competent and competitive.

Daily work provides repetition, but true mastery requires deliberate learning: reviewing new procedures, practicing instrument assembly, studying anatomy, and asking surgeons questions to deepen understanding.

Cross-training across specialties keeps your knowledge fresh and prevents stagnation. Spending time in orthopedics, neuro, robotics, ENT, or trauma challenges you and expands your competence.

Techs also participate in continuing education — conferences, workshops, webinars, and vendor demonstrations. These opportunities introduce new instruments, techniques, and evidence-based practices.

Self-assessment is crucial. After tough cases, great techs reflect:

"What went well?"

"What could I have done better?"

"What do I need to study?"

They also learn from peers, observing different setups and instrument placements.

Skill sharpness is not about perfection —

it's about consistent intention.

The best techs remain students forever.

Q79. How do Surgical Technologists decide whether to become Certified Surgical First Assistants (CSFAs)?

Becoming a CSFA is a strategic career decision that depends on passion, readiness, and professional goals. Techs consider this path when they crave deeper involvement — suturing, retracting, assisting with closure, handling tissue directly, and becoming an extension of the surgeon's hands.

The first question is motivation. Do you enjoy the technical intensity of surgery beyond instrument passing? Do you want to step closer to the operative field? Do you enjoy anatomy, precision, and advanced skills?

Second, techs assess readiness. Most CSFA programs require experience, continuing education, and strong foundational knowledge. You should feel comfortable with procedural flow, instrument mastery, and anticipation before stepping into an assist role.

Third, you evaluate your environment. Some hospitals strongly support CSFAs, using them in specialty services. Others rely more on residents or PAs. Understanding local demand matters.

Fourth, consider the lifestyle. CSFAs often earn more but may take additional call, work longer hours, or handle more physically demanding responsibilities.

Finally, talk to mentors. Ask CSFAs what they love and what they struggle with.

Becoming a CSFA is not a promotion —

it's an evolution for techs who want deeper surgical involvement.

Q80. How do Surgical Technologists develop strong professional reputations?

Your reputation follows you through every OR, every case, every interaction — and it is built through consistent excellence.

Strong reputations come from showing up early, preparing thoroughly, keeping calm under pressure, and maintaining sterile integrity at all times. Surgeons trust techs who bring predictability and precision.

You also build reputation through how you treat others. Respectful communication, willingness to help, and team-oriented behavior elevate you beyond technical skill.

Professional reputations grow through reliability. When people know you'll handle complex cases, tough surgeons, or unexpected complications without losing composure, you become invaluable.

Reputation is not built in a day.

It's built in a thousand small moments —

many no one sees but everyone feels.

Q81. How do Surgical Technologists handle ethical dilemmas in the OR?

Ethical dilemmas surface when safety, professionalism, or patient dignity feels compromised. These moments require courage.

If sterility is violated, even subtly, you must speak up. The OR is not a place for silent hesitation. You protect the patient first.

If team members behave unprofessionally, use disrespectful language, or escalate conflict, your role is to maintain calm and report concerns appropriately to leadership or charge staff.

If documentation, specimen handling, or counts appear incorrect, you bring it forward immediately.

Ethical dilemmas also include advocating for breaks, protecting new students from unsafe learning environments, and refusing to cut corners under pressure.

Your moral compass matters.

A strong ethical foundation builds trust —

and trust builds teams.

Q82. How do Surgical Technologists manage fear or anxiety when first starting out?

New techs often feel overwhelmed — and that's normal. Fear arises from the pressure to perform, the complexity of procedures, and the intensity of OR culture.

The key to managing fear is preparation. Study procedures. Practice instrument setups. Review preference cards. Take notes. Knowledge decreases anxiety.

Next, give yourself grace. No one starts confident. Even the strongest techs were once nervous beginners with shaky hands and racing hearts.

Ask questions. Seek mentorship. Shadow different techs. Watch their hands, their posture, their timing.

Use grounding techniques. Take deep breaths before scrubbing in. Use slow, deliberate motions to steady yourself.

Celebrate small wins — a clean pass, a successful count, a smooth case.

Anxiety decreases as competence increases.

Confidence comes from showing up again and again.

Q83. How do Surgical Technologists handle surgeons with very different personalities?

You might work with a surgeon who is quiet, another who is intense, another who jokes nonstop, and another who is extremely particular. Your adaptability becomes essential.

For quiet surgeons, you respond to subtle cues — hand position, body language, rhythm. You minimize verbal communication.

For intense surgeons, you maintain calm, pass instruments confidently, and avoid reacting to pressure.

For talkative surgeons, you stay professional, engaging only when appropriate while maintaining focus.

For highly particular surgeons, you study their preference cards, observe their routines, and learn their exact expectations.

The key is emotional neutrality. You adjust your style without compromising your professional identity.

Your goal isn't to change surgeons —

it's to sync with them.

Q84. What does "OR culture" mean, and why is it so important?

OR culture refers to the unspoken norms, expectations, communication patterns, hierarchies, teamwork habits, and emotional atmosphere that define the surgical environment.

It's the feeling when you walk into a room:

Is it collaborative or tense?

Respectful or chaotic?

Supportive or punitive?

OR culture influences everything — efficiency, safety, staff morale, retention, and patient outcomes.

Strong cultures value communication, respect, learning, safety, and teamwork. Weak cultures tolerate bullying, blame, ego, and silence.

Techs play a major role in shaping culture. Your tone, your professionalism, your sterile conscience, and your willingness to speak up influence the entire room.

Culture is not created by one person —

it is sustained by everyone.

Q85. Why is adaptability considered the greatest strength of a Surgical Technologist?

Because nothing in the OR stays the same. Procedures change mid-case. Surgeons shift preferences. Equipment breaks. Unexpected anatomy appears. Emergencies develop. Room assignments flip. Timelines stretch. Nights run long.

Adaptability means remaining calm in chaos. It means pivoting without panic, learning constantly, and holding yourself with quiet confidence even when variables shift.

Adaptability makes you valuable, respected, and trusted. It turns you into the tech who can handle any case, any surgeon, any scenario.

Adaptability is not flexibility —

it is mastery under changing conditions.

It is the skill that makes the OR work.

Q86. How do Surgical Technologists learn to stay calm during emergencies?

Calmness in emergencies isn't something you're born with — it's a skill you develop through exposure, mentorship, and internal discipline. The first time an emergency hits the OR, your heart races. You feel the tension in the air, the urgency in the surgeon's voice, the quick steps of anesthesia. But the more emergencies you experience, the more you understand that the room needs stability — and you can provide it.

Calmness begins with preparation. When you know your instruments, know your backup plans, and know where everything lives, your brain stays grounded even when chaos pulses around you. Surprises don't feel like surprises — they feel like deviations you were ready to handle.

The next layer is controlled breathing. Even one slow breath resets your nervous system and prevents panic from taking over your hands. Many experienced techs rely on this technique silently throughout emergencies.

You also draw strength from the team. The OR becomes a hive mind in crisis: anesthesia stabilizing vitals, circulators opening more supplies, surgeons acting decisively. You plug into that collective focus. You become part of the solution.

Finally, calmness comes from purpose. You're not just passing instruments — you're helping save a life. When you anchor yourself in that truth, clarity overcomes fear.

Emergencies don't get easier.

You get stronger.

Q87. How do Surgical Technologists handle the physical demands of the job?

This profession is physically taxing. You stand for hours, often locked into one position. You hold retractors with steady force. You push heavy equipment. You move trays that weigh more than you expect. You pivot, reach, bend, lift, and stretch.

Surgical Technologists manage this through intentional physical habits. Good posture becomes a daily discipline — shoulders relaxed, back straight, knees slightly bent. You learn to shift your weight during long cases to prevent fatigue. You wear supportive shoes and compression socks. Some techs use insoles or rotate pairs during the week.

Stretching becomes essential. Techs often stretch before cases, during turnovers, and after shifts. Simple movements — rolling shoulders, flexing wrists, rotating hips — preserve longevity.

Hydration matters. Fatigue increases dramatically when you're dehydrated. Quick sips during turnovers add up.

Strength training helps too. Strong core muscles protect your back when lifting trays or assisting with patient positioning. Even light dumbbells or resistance bands at home can improve endurance.

Finally, techs listen to their bodies. Pain is information, not a weakness. Adjusting technique, asking for help lifting, or taking a moment to reset prevents long-term injury.

You don't endure the physical demands of this job by accident —

you endure them by caring for the vessel that carries your skill.

Q88. What does it mean when surgeons request a specific tech by name?

When surgeons request you by name, it means you've crossed an invisible threshold: you're no longer just part of the team — you're part of *their* surgical identity.

Surgeons value predictability, rhythm, and trust. When they request you, they're saying:

- "You enhance my performance."
- "You anticipate my needs."

- "You make my cases smoother."
- "I trust you with my patient — and my reputation."

This is one of the highest compliments in the OR. It means your sterile technique is impeccable, your anticipation is sharp, your energy stabilizes the room, and your setups match their style perfectly.

But it also brings responsibility. Requested techs often handle difficult cases, challenging patients, complex reconstructions, and longer procedures. Your reputation becomes an asset for the entire OR.

When you're requested, protect that trust. Keep learning. Stay humble. Show the same consistency that earned you the recognition.

When a surgeon says, "I want them on my case,"

it means you've become irreplaceable in that moment —

and unforgettable in their practice.

Q89. How do Surgical Technologists balance speed and accuracy during rapid-fire cases?

Some OR days move at lightning speed — short cases, fast turnovers, surgeons with high energy, and schedules stacked tightly. Surgical Technologists must master the art of moving quickly *without* compromising accuracy, sterility, or safety.

Speed begins long before the case starts. You study preference cards, pull supplies early, label sutures, and organize your back table for maximum efficiency. Proper preparation eliminates 80% of delays.

During rapid-fire cases, your movements stay smooth — not jerky. You pass instruments cleanly, retract confidently, and handle sutures without tangling. The faster the case moves, the quieter your energy becomes.

Accuracy comes from mindfulness. Even in short cases, counts must be flawless. Sterility must remain uncompromised. Documentation must be correct. You cannot let pace undermine precision.

Communication strengthens both speed and accuracy. Brief, clear statements like "Knife up," "Next suture ready," and "Camera switch" keep the room aligned.

When speed and accuracy coexist, the OR feels like a seamless machine — and you become one of its most valuable gears.

Q90. How do Surgical Technologists help create a supportive environment for new graduates?

New grads enter the OR wide-eyed, anxious, hopeful, and overwhelmed. A supportive environment is built not through grand gestures, but through a thousand tiny kindnesses and shared knowledge.

You set the tone with patience. You explain setups piece by piece. You encourage questions. You normalize mistakes as part of learning. You share tips and tricks: how to fold a gown quickly, how to organize a Mayo stand, how to stay calm during intense moments.

Support also means protecting them from unrealistic expectations. You reassure them that no one is expected to know everything on day one. You remind them that confidence comes with repetition.

You model professionalism. You demonstrate sterile conscience, respect for teammates, and emotional steadiness.

You celebrate their small wins. Completing a clean count. Setting up a room independently. Passing instruments smoothly for the first time.

A healthy OR grows its own.

Supporting new grads strengthens the future of your profession.

Q91. What should Surgical Technologists understand about elective vs emergency surgeries?

Elective surgeries run on predictability. Emergency surgeries run on adrenaline.

Elective cases have clear plans, scheduled times, familiar instruments, and calm pacing. You have time to prep trays, read preference cards, and organize a meticulous setup. Patients are usually medically optimized.

Emergency surgeries are the opposite. They arrive unannounced, often with incomplete information and rapidly deteriorating conditions. You may not have every detail. The team improvises within protocol. Speed matters, but safety cannot be sacrificed.

Techs must shift gears instantly. Your hands must be steady even when the room feels urgent. Your anticipation becomes sharper, your communication cleaner, and your awareness heightened.

Both types of surgeries require excellence –

but emergencies reveal the depth of your training and the strength of your composure.

Q92. What makes the OR such a unique work environment compared to other healthcare settings?

The OR is unlike any environment in healthcare. It is intensely technical, emotionally charged, and deeply ritualistic.

It's a place where silence has meaning, urgency has rhythm, and teamwork has choreography. Every movement matters. Every second matters. Every role matters.

The OR blends science, art, and instinct. You work inches from the body's secrets: anatomy exposed, pathology revealed, healing enacted in real time.

Unlike other hospital units, the OR is closed to the public. It operates as its own hidden world with its own culture, language, rules, and hierarchy. You bond with your team through shared stress, shared victories, and shared responsibility.

The OR demands excellence and rewards mastery. It challenges your mind, body, and emotions. It forces growth and resilience. It gives you moments of awe you never forget.

The OR is not just a workplace –

it's a calling and a community.

Q93. How do Surgical Technologists build confidence over time?

Confidence comes slowly, quietly, and through repetition. It's not a sudden switch — it's a gradual strengthening.

It begins when you stop memorizing steps and start understanding them. When instruments stop being shapes and start being tools with purpose. When surgeons' movements become familiar. When emergencies no longer shake your core.

Confidence builds each time you handle a difficult case and stay composed. Each time you adapt to a new specialty. Each time you catch a potential error. Each time a surgeon nods with approval. Each time a coworker says, "I'm glad you're in this room with me."

You don't become confident by avoiding mistakes —

you become confident by learning from them.

Confidence is earned slowly, but once it arrives, it becomes your anchor.

Q94. How do Surgical Technologists stay motivated on tough days?

Motivation isn't constant. Some days the cases are long, the room is tense, the turnover is heavy, or the emotional load hits hard. Techs stay motivated by reconnecting with purpose.

You remember the patients — the real humans behind each incision. You remember the moments where your work mattered: stopping bleeding, preventing contamination, saving someone's life.

You draw motivation from your team. The OR is family —

flawed, imperfect, but fiercely united. Their strength fuels yours.

You also find motivation in mastery. Each day refines your skill. Each challenge sharpens your edge. Each setback deepens your experience.

And on the hardest days, you remind yourself:

You are part of something bigger than the struggle.

The OR is not easy —

but it is meaningful.

And meaning sustains motivation.

Q95. Why do Surgical Technologists often feel protective of the sterile field?

Because the sterile field is sacred. It is where trust lives. It is where patients are safest. It is where your hands become their shield against infection, complications, and harm.

Techs feel protective because they build the field themselves. They drape it, guard it, maintain it, and repair it when needed. It becomes an extension of their professional identity.

A break in sterility can change a patient's life. Techs know this, feel this, and carry this responsibility deeply.

Protecting the sterile field is not controlling —

it is caring.

It is the purest expression of a Surgical Technologist's calling.

Q96. How do Surgical Technologists recover after a mentally draining shift?

Recovery is essential for longevity. After mentally draining shifts, techs decompress intentionally.

Some use quiet rituals: driving home in silence, taking a long shower, sitting outside, listening to calming music. Others use connection: talking to coworkers, sharing the story of the day, or calling a loved one.

Physical release matters too — stretching, walking, exercising, or simply lying down and letting the body unwind.

Journaling helps process emotional weight. So does humor. So does rest.

Recovery is not weakness.

It is maintenance of your humanity.

Q97. What does growth look like for a Surgical Technologist who chooses not to specialize?

Not all techs specialize — and those who don't still grow tremendously. Generalists become Swiss Army knives of the OR: adaptable, knowledgeable, confident in a wide range of procedures.

Growth looks like mastering multiple services: general surgery, gynecology, urology, ENT, plastics, vascular, and more. It looks like becoming the tech leadership calls when a case needs someone competent in anything.

Generalists become mentors, educators, preceptors, and often charge techs. They maintain broad knowledge and refine efficiency across specialties.

Choosing not to specialize is not limiting —

it's expanding.

Q98. How does a Surgical Technologist know they've truly "made it" in the OR?

The moment varies for everyone, but common milestones include:

- The first time you anticipate every step in a case
- The first time a surgeon says, "Great job today"
- The first time you catch an error before anyone else
- The first time you handle a trauma without shaking
- The first time you realize you're not thinking — you're *flowing*
- The first time someone requests you for their room
- The first time a student says, "I want to be like you"

You know you've made it when the OR no longer feels intimidating —

it feels like home.

Q99. What keeps Surgical Technologists in the profession long-term?

Many stay because they love the pace, the challenge, the camaraderie, and the meaning. They love the adrenaline, the precision, the teamwork, and the artistry of surgery.

Some stay because they continually evolve — moving into education, leadership, specialty roles, or assisting.

Most stay because the OR becomes part of who they are. The rhythms, the routines, the rituals — they imprint on you.

People don't stay for the job.

They stay for the calling.

Q100. What makes Surgical Technology a career worth choosing today?

Because few careers offer the blend of purpose, skill, stability, growth, and impact that Surgical Technology does.

You enter a field where your hands matter, your voice matters, your vigilance matters. You become part of life-saving moments, high-tech innovations, and deeply human experiences.

You gain a career with mobility, specialization options, competitive pay, and national demand. You join a community built on excellence, courage, and resilience.

Surgical Technology is not an easy path —

but it is a meaningful one.

And for those who are called to the OR,

there is no better place to be.

Q101. "If I'm being completely honest with myself, should I become a Surgical Technologist — or would another path fit me better?"

This question is not about whether you *can* do the job. Many people are capable of learning the technical skills required for the operating room. The real question is whether the daily rhythm of this work — standing for long procedures, working in high-precision environments, functioning within surgical team hierarchies, and maintaining constant attention to sterile detail — feels sustainable for you over time.

Take a moment to reflect on what you have learned throughout this guide. Which Day-in-the-Life stories felt energizing rather than draining? Which responsibilities felt meaningful rather than heavy? Which environments seemed to match your pace, personality, and tolerance for pressure?

If you can picture yourself doing this work repeatedly and still feeling a sense of purpose, focus, and professional pride, Surgical Technology may be a strong alignment. If the role consistently feels tense, exhausting, or mismatched with the life you want to build, it does not mean you failed — it means you gained clarity. Alignment is not about choosing the most impressive path; it is about choosing the path you can live inside, day after day, without slowly burning out.

Chapter 12

Salary Guide and Job Market Outlook

Surgical Technology is one of the few healthcare careers where salary, demand, and mobility come together in a way that gives professionals real leverage. The operating room (OR) is the financial engine of the hospital, and the people who keep it running are consistently in short supply. This guide gives future Surgical Technologists a clear, honest look at where the money is, where shortages exist, and how to maximize long-term earning power in this profession.

1. Understanding the Surgical Technologist Salary Landscape

Surgical Technologists sit at a unique point in the healthcare pay spectrum. You are not compensated at the level of physicians or nurse anesthetists, yet your skill set is specialized enough that hospitals cannot function without you. That scarcity directly influences earnings. National wages continue to rise as OR volume grows and staffing shortages intensify. Salary reflects the complexity of surgery, the need for trained hands, the cost of surgical delays, regional shortages, and the surgical case mix in a given market. When a Surgical Technologist is missing, cases cannot start. When turnover slows, surgeons lose productivity. When new technology arrives, techs must master it. These realities push salaries higher not out of generosity, but necessity.

2. Highest-Paying States for Surgical Technologists

Some states pay significantly more due to shortages, cost of living, rural access issues, surgical volume, and aggressive health-system competition for talent. Top-paying states typically include:

1 **California** — High cost of living, dense surgical volume, and union influence in some regions drive strong compensation; travel ST pay is especially high.

2 **Alaska** — Remote access and persistent staffing shortages maintain elevated rates.

3 **Washington & Oregon** — High acuity case mix and system competition for experienced techs.

4 **Massachusetts, Connecticut, New York** — High concentration of academic medical centers performing complex surgical care.

5 **Colorado & Nevada** — Rapid population growth fueling expanding surgical demand.

6 **Texas** — Extremely high surgical volume and rapid hospital expansion create abundant opportunity.

7 **Florida** — Large orthopedic, cardiac, ENT, and robotics volumes drive competitive metro-area pay.

3. Highest-Paying Cities for OR Work

Large cities and high-volume surgical corridors pay more, especially where multiple health systems compete, trauma centers require experienced staff, outpatient surgical networks are large, and robotics or orthopedic caseloads are heavy. Examples include Los Angeles, the San Francisco Bay Area, Seattle, Boston, New York City, Houston, Dallas, Austin, San Antonio, Denver, Miami, Tampa, and Orlando. These markets also attract travel techs, which further drives wage competition.

4. Highest-Paying Specialties for Surgical Technologists

Specialty equals leverage. Hospitals pay more to recruit techs who master demanding service lines:

1 **Cardiothoracic Surgery** — Complex sequencing, bypass equipment, and delicate tissue work.

2 **Neurosurgery** — Long-duration cases requiring precision and micro-instrument expertise.

3 **Orthopedics (Trauma & Joint Replacement)** — Heavy trays, implants, and power tools requiring stamina and technical familiarity.

4 **Robotics** — Troubleshooting systems, docking robotic arms, and managing specialized instrumentation.

5 **Vascular Surgery** — High-risk cases involving grafts, clamps, and delicate suturing.

6 **OB/GYN High-Risk Surgery** — Emergent procedures and neonatal-support coordination.

5. Where the Biggest Shortages Are Right Now

Shortages appear in several consistent areas:

1 Rural hospitals — Often offer relocation bonuses, loan repayment, higher base pay, and flexible scheduling to recruit staff.

2 Large trauma centers — Volume, acuity, and burnout create constant openings.

3 Outpatient surgery centers (ASCs) — Rapid expansion has intensified competition for experienced techs.

4 Teaching hospitals — Slower case flow makes experienced techs especially valuable.

5 High-growth states — Nevada, Arizona, Texas, Florida, Utah, and Tennessee continue to show strong demand.

6. Travel Surgical Technologist Pay

Travel assignments significantly increase earning potential. Many travel Surgical Technologists earn double local pay depending on crisis rates, specialty shortages, geographic demand, and night or holiday incentives. Typical reports include $1,800–$2,400 weekly take-home, $2,800–$3,500 weekly for high-demand contracts, and even higher during crisis staffing periods or in remote regions. Travel work is not for everyone, but for some it accelerates savings, debt repayment, and financial flexibility.

7. How Shift Differentials Add Thousands Each Year

Evening, night, and weekend differentials are often overlooked income boosters. Evening shifts may add $1–$3 per hour, nights $2–$6 per hour, and weekends $3–$10 per hour. Strategic scheduling around these differentials can increase annual income by $5,000–$12,000 without changing employers.

8. On-Call Pay: A Hidden Income Source

On-call programs frequently include hourly stipends, overtime when called in, and time-and-a-half or double-time for holidays. Call-heavy specialties such as trauma, orthopedic, neuro, vascular, and cardiac surgery can add thousands annually. Some techs significantly increase income by stacking call strategically.

9. How to Negotiate a Surgical Technologist Salary

Negotiation is often underused. Strong specialty skills in orthopedics, robotics, neuro, or cardiac surgery create leverage. Bring market data, demonstrate how your skills prevent delays, leverage competing offers when possible, and negotiate beyond base pay. Sign-on bonuses, relocation assistance, additional differentials, guaranteed hours, call structure, and scheduling flexibility are all negotiable elements. Thoughtful negotiation can raise total compensation 10–20 percent immediately.

10. The Future Job Outlook for Surgical Technologists

Rising surgical volume, an aging population, expanding robotics, increasing outpatient procedures, and nationwide OR staffing shortages continue to drive demand. Official projections suggest roughly 5–7 percent job growth, but many high-scarcity regions experience demand that feels closer to 15–20 percent. As robotics expands, ASCs multiply, surgeons increase weekly case loads, and turnover efficiency becomes more critical, the need for highly trained Surgical Technologists will continue to rise. This is not a fading career; it is a growing one.

11. The Bottom Line: Where You Earn the Most

To maximize income, focus on high-paying regions (West Coast, Northeast, Mountain West), high-paying specialties (cardiac, orthopedic, neuro, robotics), high-paying settings (trauma centers, ASCs, major surgical corridors), high-earning structures (travel contracts, night shifts, call-heavy roles), and strong negotiation strategies based on scarcity rather than years of experience.

Chapter 13

Fit Analyzer™

Surgical Technologist Role Fit Index (RFI)

If the Mini SCRUB*fit*™ Healthcare Career Assessment helped you explore whether healthcare broadly fits you, the Role Fit Index below helps you evaluate something more specific: whether the Surgical Technologist role itself matches how you naturally work.

The Surgical Technologist role is built around precision, rhythm, anticipation, and steady performance under pressure. Some people feel immediately energized inside the operating room environment, while others discover that the pace, sensory demands, or physical structure of the work feels heavier than expected. The purpose of this Fit Analyzer™ is not to determine whether you *can* do the job — many people can. The goal is to help you understand whether the environment naturally fits how you are wired.

Read each statement below and rate how true it feels for you using the following scale:

1 = Not at all true for me

5 = Sometimes true for me

10 = Extremely true for me

Write your number next to each statement and total your score at the end.

Role Fit Index Statements

1. I enjoy work that requires precision and attention to small details.

2. I can remain focused for long periods without becoming mentally restless.

3. Fast-paced environments feel energizing rather than overwhelming to me.

4. I am comfortable following structured procedures and established sequences.

5. I like anticipating what others need before they ask for it.

6. Standing for long periods or working physically demanding shifts does not bother me.

7. I stay calm when unexpected problems occur.

8. I prefer team-based environments where each person has a defined role.

9. I am comfortable working in environments with bright lights, noise, and constant activity.

10. I take pride in supporting outcomes even when my role is mostly behind the scenes.

11. I enjoy learning specialized tools, instruments, or technical systems.

12. I can accept direct feedback or fast corrections without taking them personally.

13. I like environments where timing, rhythm, and coordination matter.

14. I am comfortable working around medical procedures or surgical settings.

15. I recover quickly after stressful situations and return to focus without difficulty.

Scoring Your RFI

Add your numbers to calculate your total score (maximum = 150).

120–150 — Strong Alignment

Your natural preferences strongly match the structure, pace, and teamwork dynamics of the operating room. You are likely to feel comfortable developing mastery in this role and may adapt quickly to specialty environments.

90–119 — Good Alignment

Many aspects of the Surgical Technologist role fit your working style. Your long-term satisfaction will often depend on choosing the right surgical specialty, schedule structure, and team environment.

60–89 — Partial Alignment

You may succeed in the role, but certain elements — pace, physical demands, or sensory intensity — could feel heavier over time. Exploring different surgical settings or adjacent technical healthcare roles may help you identify the best long-term fit.

Below 60 — Potential Misalignment

The operating room environment may not match your natural energy patterns or preferred working conditions. Healthcare still offers many strong pathways where your strengths may feel more sustainable and rewarding.

Reflection

Your score is not a label. It is a signal — a starting point for reflection. As you read the Day-in-the-Life chapters and explore the experiences of different Surgical Technologists, notice which environments feel energizing, which feel neutral, and which feel draining. Those reactions often tell you more about long-term career sustainability than any test score alone.

The goal of the **SCRUB*fit*™** approach is simple: help you find the healthcare environment where your wiring, your pace, and your purpose naturally align — before you commit years of training to a role that may not fit.

Chapter 14

Surgical Technologist Specialty Guide

How Different OR Worlds Shape Your Skills, Your Pay, and Your Identity

One of the greatest advantages of becoming a Surgical Technologist is that you do not simply choose a career — you choose a specialty universe. Each specialty feels like its own surgical culture, with its own pace, rituals, sounds, personalities, and emotional gravity. Some specialties demand endurance, some demand micro-precision, some demand speed, and some demand extraordinary calm. All demand excellence. This chapter offers a clear, cinematic look at what each specialty feels like from the inside — the challenges, the opportunities, the pay advantages, and the personality fit that makes one environment feel like home.

1. Orthopedic Surgery: The Kingdom of Steel, Power Tools, and Adrenaline

If you love mechanics, structure, and the satisfying click of metal meeting bone, orthopedics may feel natural. Orthopedic surgery is physical, fast, and full of heavy trays — bone saws, drills, reduction clamps (gl), plates, rods, and implants. Joint replacements require precision, trauma cases bring controlled chaos, sports medicine demands speed, and spine surgery requires stamina and meticulous sequencing. Orthopedic techs are valued for memorizing tray layouts, anticipating implant sizing, managing vendors, and keeping pace with surgeons who work quickly. This is one of the highest-paying specialties because experienced orthopedic techs are consistently in demand.

2. Neurosurgery: The Symphony of Stillness

Neurosurgery operates on a microscopic scale using delicate dissectors, ultra-fine forceps, bipolar cautery (gl), and sutures so small they resemble threads of silk. Neuro techs must master patience, controlled movement, micro-instrumentation, and sustained focus during long cases such as craniotomies (gl), tumor resections (gl), and aneurysm repairs (gl). The specialty offers deep trust, technical prestige, and some of the longest, most intense procedures in the OR.

3. Cardiothoracic Surgery: Where the Heart Defines the Tempo

Cardiac surgery is precise, highly coordinated work involving sternal saws, bypass equipment (gl), grafts (gl), and magnified suturing. Surgical technologists collaborate closely with perfusionists (gl), specialized anesthesia teams, and cardiothoracic surgeons. Because these skills are rare and the stakes are high, compensation in this specialty is often elevated.

4. Trauma Surgery: The Art of Controlled Urgency

Trauma cases include emergent laparotomies (gl), severe injuries, and vascular emergencies requiring immediate preparation and rapid anticipation. Trauma techs develop strong problem-solving skills, equipment mastery across specialties, and emotional resilience after difficult outcomes. These professionals are highly respected for remaining steady when seconds matter.

5. Robotics: The Future-Facing Specialty

Robotic surgery continues expanding rapidly. Surgical technologists trained in robotic systems learn docking procedures, robotic instrumentation, system troubleshooting, and equipment calibration. Because relatively few techs master these skills, robotic specialists often gain additional influence and negotiating leverage.

6. Gynecology & Women's Health Surgery

Gynecologic surgery blends delicate anatomy with strong surgical pacing. Techs work with laparoscopic (gl) equipment, pelvic reconstructive devices, and energy platforms (gl). Teams in this specialty often develop tight working relationships built on trust and clinical coordination.

7. Labor & Delivery / C-Section Surgery

Cesarean section rooms combine surgical precision with the emotional intensity of childbirth. Surgical technologists prepare neonatal supplies (gl), emergency hemorrhage setups (gl), and standard C-section trays while supporting both mother and infant during rapidly evolving situations.

8. ENT (Ear, Nose, Throat): The World of Small Spaces

ENT procedures rely on delicate instrumentation, laser safety protocols (gl), and airway-focused surgical workflows. This specialty blends speed with finesse and suits techs who enjoy detailed work and frequent case turnover.

9. Plastics & Reconstructive Surgery: The Artistry Specialty

Plastic surgery combines surgical science with aesthetic reconstruction. Cases may include microsurgery (gl), burn reconstruction, hand surgery, and facial reconstruction. Surgical technologists develop expertise in graft preparation (gl), delicate retraction, and specialized instrumentation.

10. Vascular Surgery: The Dance of Blood Flow

Vascular surgery involves graft placement, clamps, microvascular suturing (gl), and endovascular (gl) tools such as guidewires and balloon systems. Precision timing and careful sequencing are critical to patient safety.

11. Urology: High-Tech, High-Precision Surgery

Urology blends robotics, endoscopic procedures (gl), and laser technology. Techs work with camera systems, irrigation devices, laser fibers, and specialty scopes during procedures such as prostatectomies (gl) and nephrectomies (gl). This specialty appeals to techs who enjoy technology-driven workflows.

12. Ophthalmology: Surgery Under a Microscope

Ophthalmic surgery involves extremely small instruments, lens implantation sets (gl), and microscope-assisted procedures. The environment is quiet, precise, and highly controlled, rewarding steady hands and patience.

13. General Surgery: The Universal Foundation

General surgery remains the backbone of the OR, covering appendectomies (gl), hernia repairs (gl), bowel resections (gl), gallbladder removal (gl), and emergency exploratory procedures. This specialty builds foundational instrumentation knowledge, sterile discipline, and adaptability that support every other surgical area.

14. Why Choosing a Specialty Matters

Specialty selection shapes earning potential, stress exposure, career stability, negotiation leverage, surgeon relationships, and professional identity. Some technologists remain in one specialty for decades, while others rotate across multiple services; both paths build mastery.

15. The Bottom Line: Specialization Creates Power

Specialization strengthens bargaining power, increases salary potential, expands travel opportunities, deepens clinical confidence, and opens doors to advanced roles such as CSTFA (Certified Surgical Technologist First Assistant) (gl). Most importantly, specialization transforms the career from a routine job into a skilled professional craft.

Chapter 15

Certification and Licensure Guide

How to Earn Your Credential, Keep It Current, and Build a Career With Staying Power

Becoming a Surgical Technologist is not only about learning how to pass instruments, maintain the sterile field (gl), or anticipate a surgeon's next move. It is about building a professional foundation strong enough to carry you through decades of operating room evolution, new technologies, specialty changes, and career growth. Certification is more than a test. It becomes your credibility, your bargaining power, your protection, and your passport into nearly every operating room in the United States. This chapter walks step by step through the journey—from training to credentialing to renewal—and explains why certification matters now more than ever.

1. The Path to Becoming a Certified Surgical Technologist (CST)

Most employers prefer, and many require, the Certified Surgical Technologist (CST) credential offered through the

National Board of Surgical Technology and Surgical Assisting (NBSTSA) (gl). The path begins with completing an accredited educational program. To sit for the CST exam, students must graduate from a program accredited by either the Commission on Accreditation of Allied Health Education Programs (CAAHEP) (gl) or the Accrediting Bureau of Health Education Schools (ABHES) (gl). These programs include classroom instruction, lab practice, sterile technique training, surgical instrumentation, surgical anatomy, and clinical rotations (gl) in real operating room environments. Competence develops through repeated real-case exposure until anticipation becomes instinct.

2. What the CST Exam Actually Tests

The CST exam measures real operating room competence. It focuses on perioperative care (gl), intraoperative care (gl), and postoperative responsibilities (gl). Topics include preparing the operating room, patient positioning, draping, surgical counts, specimen handling (gl), instrument identification, maintaining the sterile field, assisting surgeons, troubleshooting equipment, instrument decontamination, turnover procedures, and documentation. The exam consists of 175 questions (150 scored and 25 unscored), is computer-based, and is administered at PSI testing centers nationwide. Passing indicates that the technologist is prepared for safe clinical practice.

3. TS-C vs. CST: What's the Difference?

Two national credentials exist. The CST (Certified Surgical Technologist) credential, issued by NBSTSA, is widely considered the gold standard and is required or strongly preferred by most employers. The TS-C (Tech in Surgery

Certified), issued by the National Center for Competency Testing (NCCT) (gl), is accepted in many facilities but not universally. While both credentials demonstrate competence, CST certification generally provides stronger mobility between states and greater negotiating leverage.

4. State-by-State Rules (Why This Matters)

Unlike some healthcare professions, Surgical Technologists do not operate under a single national licensure system. Some states require certification for practice, others require accredited education and demonstrated competency, and some allow hospital-level requirements to determine hiring standards. Even in states without formal regulation, certification is strongly preferred because it reduces institutional risk and supports patient safety.

5. How to Prepare for the CST Exam Without Overwhelm

Preparation becomes manageable when approached in layers. First, build core knowledge of sterile technique, instrumentation, anatomy, and case sequencing. Second, complete structured practice tests to understand pacing and question formats. Third, connect study topics to real clinical experiences gained during rotations. Finally, memorize instruments strategically by linking each tool to its purpose, specialty, and point of use during procedures.

6. How Long Certification Lasts (and How Renewal Works)

The CST credential must be renewed every four years. Renewal typically occurs through completion of 60 continuing education (CE) credits (gl), earned through conferences, workshops, specialty courses, vendor education, online modules, or in-service (gl) training. Continuing education ensures that technologists remain current with robotic systems, new implants, evolving sterile standards, and specialty innovations. Re-testing is also an option, although less commonly chosen.

7. How Certification Impacts Salary, Hiring, and Mobility

Certification significantly influences career value. Certified technologists are associated with reduced surgical errors, improved efficiency, stronger sterile technique adherence, and faster adaptation to complex cases. Certified Surgical Technologists often earn several dollars more per hour than non-certified peers and qualify for a broader range of travel contracts and specialty roles.

8. Additional Certifications for Career Growth

After establishing experience, technologists can pursue additional credentials. Certified Surgical First Assistant (CSFA) (gl) certification allows expanded intraoperative responsibilities such as tissue handling, suturing, retraction, and incision closure. Robotic surgery certification provides specialization in advanced surgical systems used across multiple specialties. Vendor-sponsored training programs in orthopedic, spine, and cardiovascular instrumentation can also strengthen technical expertise and professional value.

9. How New Technologists Use Certification to Stand Out During Hiring

New graduates often underestimate their leverage. Certification signals professionalism, baseline competence, readiness for complex procedures, and long-term commitment to the profession. Hiring managers, charge nurses, and surgical teams frequently prioritize certified applicants because they require less training and integrate more quickly into clinical workflow.

10. The Emotional Meaning of Earning Your Credential

Passing the CST exam represents more than academic achievement. It marks the transition from student to professional—from learning the field to actively protecting it. Certification reflects commitment, discipline, and readiness for responsibility. For many technologists, the moment they receive confirmation of certification becomes a defining milestone: the moment they step into the operating room not as trainees, but as trusted members of the surgical team.

Chapter 16

Travel Surgical Technologist Master Guide

How to Multiply Your Income, Expand Your Skills, and See the Country — One Operating Room at a Time

There is a moment in many Surgical Technologists' careers when the operating room begins to feel deeply familiar. Your hands know every instrument. Your surgeons know your rhythm. Your rooms feel predictable. Then you hear about travel technologists—about the pay, the mobility, and the opportunity to work across the country one contract at a time. Traveling as a Surgical Technologist is not a vacation; it is a professional transformation that expands your earning power, your clinical exposure, and your professional identity. This chapter serves as a practical roadmap for understanding how travel assignments work and how they can reshape a career.

1. What Travel Surgical Technologists Actually Do

Travel technologists work short-term contracts—typically 8, 13, or 26 weeks—at hospitals and ambulatory surgery centers (ASC) (gl) experiencing staffing shortages, expansion, or seasonal surgical demand. Their role is to maintain operating room efficiency, assist in specialties where they already have experience, adapt quickly with minimal orientation, and support teams during staffing surges or turnover periods.

2. Why the Pay Is So High (And Why It Remains Strong)

Hospitals pay premium rates for travel technologists because surgical services generate a major portion of hospital revenue. When operating rooms close or cases are delayed due to staffing shortages, financial losses occur immediately. Travel technologists fill these critical gaps. Compensation packages typically include hourly pay, tax-advantaged housing stipends, meal per diem (gl), overtime eligibility, call pay, and completion bonuses. Specialty technologists in orthopedics, cardiothoracic, neurosurgery, trauma, or robotics often command the highest compensation.

3. Regions With the Highest Demand

Demand fluctuates based on population growth, regional shortages, and surgical volume. States such as California, Washington, Oregon, Colorado, Alaska, Texas, Arizona, Nevada, Florida, New York, and Massachusetts frequently offer strong contract availability. Traveling allows professionals to choose assignments based on income goals, geographic preference, seasonal lifestyle, or specialty experience.

4. Choosing the Right Travel Agency

Travel agencies significantly influence the traveler's experience. Important evaluation factors include transparent compensation breakdowns, recruiter responsiveness, agency reputation with hospitals, clinical support availability, contract clarity, and the breadth of available job listings. Many experienced travelers maintain relationships with multiple agencies to expand contract options and negotiating leverage.

5. Negotiating Travel Contracts Effectively

Negotiation strength depends on specialty expertise, geographic flexibility, willingness to accept evening or weekend schedules, call availability, and rapid-response readiness. Assignments requiring short-notice start dates or service in underserved regions often offer the highest compensation.

6. Contract Red Flags to Watch For

Travelers should review contracts carefully for unclear call expectations, floating requirements outside core specialties, unpaid orientation time, low guaranteed weekly hours, or unsafe staffing ratios. A reliable recruiter should explain each contract component in detail and advise when an assignment may not be a good fit.

7. Housing and Financial Strategy

Housing stipends often represent a large portion of travel compensation. Many travelers secure furnished apartments, extended-stay housing, short-term rentals, or RV accommodations to maintain housing expenses below the stipend amount, allowing the difference to contribute directly to savings.

8. Orientation Expectations

Orientation periods are typically brief and focused on facility onboarding, electronic health record (EHR) (gl) access, department workflow, and preference card (gl) review. Travelers are expected to function independently soon after arrival, applying existing specialty expertise while adapting to local workflows.

9. How Travel Work Accelerates Skill Development

Travel assignments expose technologists to multiple surgical cultures, instrumentation systems, surgeon preferences, documentation workflows, and equipment environments. This diversity of exposure rapidly strengthens adaptability, clinical judgment, and technical versatility.

10. Professional Behaviors That Support Travel Success

Successful travelers demonstrate adaptability, humility, strong communication, rapid learning ability, emotional composure, and respect for local team dynamics. The ability to integrate quickly into unfamiliar environments is often the defining factor in repeat contract requests.

11. Understanding Different Operating Room Cultures

Operating rooms differ widely in pace, communication style, hierarchy, and workflow. Some environments emphasize speed and high-volume turnover, while others prioritize highly structured academic workflows. Travel technologists develop the skill of quickly assessing team rhythm and adapting their communication and work style accordingly.

12. Personal and Professional Growth Through Travel

Travel assignments frequently expand professional confidence, resilience, independence, networking opportunities, and financial stability. Exposure to diverse clinical environments encourages broader clinical competence and leadership readiness.

13. When to Begin Traveling

Most technologists begin traveling after approximately 18–24 months of core specialty experience, once sterile technique confidence, case sequencing familiarity, and independent functioning skills are firmly established.

14. Using Travel Work as a Financial Strategy

Travel assignments can accelerate financial goals such as student loan repayment, home purchasing, emergency savings growth, investment building, or funding additional education such as surgical first assisting programs. For many professionals, travel work becomes a strategic income accelerator rather than a permanent employment model.

15. The Bottom Line: Expanding Your Surgical World

Traveling broadens professional perspective by exposing technologists to rural hospitals, urban trauma centers, academic teaching institutions, outpatient surgical environments, and specialty-focused facilities. This exposure builds adaptability, strengthens clinical mastery, and often transforms confident technologists into recognized leaders within surgical services.

Chapter 17

Résumé Prep for Surgical Technologists

How to Present Your Technical Skills, OR Experience, and Professional Readiness Clearly and Confidently

A Surgical Technologist's résumé must accomplish two essential goals: communicate your technical competence in the operating room and demonstrate your ability to function effectively in one of the most high-stakes environments in healthcare. Unlike many clinical roles, the Surgical Technologist résumé is not about lengthy narrative; it is about precision, safety, clarity, and proof that you can anticipate the needs of the surgical team. This chapter provides a clean, modern résumé blueprint designed specifically for Surgical Technologists entering, advancing within, or relocating across the operating room landscape.

Part I: The Purpose of a Surgical Technologist Résumé

Your résumé is not a career diary; it is a readability test. When a Surgical Services Manager scans your résumé, they are looking for four immediate answers: Can you function safely and confidently in their operating room? Which specialties and service lines can you scrub in? How quickly can you onboard? Do you understand sterile technique, instrumentation, workflow, and surgical priorities? Your résumé should answer these questions instantly.

Part II: The Gold-Standard Surgical Technologist Résumé Structure

1. Header and Credentials

List your name followed immediately by credentials if applicable (for example: Alex Rivera, CST). Include phone number, professional email address, city and state, and LinkedIn profile if available.

2. Professional Summary (3–4 sentences)

Provide a concise snapshot of your professional identity. Include years of experience, core specialties, primary strengths such as anticipation, instrumentation expertise, sterile technique, and turnover efficiency, and your approach to teamwork and patient safety.

Example: Surgical Technologist with four years of experience supporting high-volume general, orthopedic, and OB/GYN surgical services. Known for precise instrumentation preparation, strong situational awareness, and the ability to anticipate surgeon needs. Recognized for meticulous sterile technique and collaborative teamwork that supports safe and efficient patient care.

3. Core Competencies (10–14 items)

This section is critical for résumé-screening systems and hiring managers. Include competencies such as sterile technique, instrumentation and equipment setup, case cart assembly, preference card management, anticipation of procedural steps, operating room workflow and turnover, laparoscopic equipment setup, surgical counts, aseptic field maintenance, specimen handling, pre-operative room preparation, post-operative breakdown, robotics support, or endoscopy support. List only skills you genuinely perform.

4. Certification and Licensure

Include CST certification (NBSTSA), BLS/CPR certification, applicable state licensure, and any additional credentials such as surgical assisting certification if applicable.

5. Education

List your Surgical Technology certificate or associate degree first, followed by additional degrees or relevant continuing education.

6. Clinical or Professional Experience

For each role, include job title, organization, location, employment dates, specialties covered, approximate case volume, and key responsibilities.

Example bullet points:

- Prepared operating rooms and surgical instruments for 15–20 procedures weekly across general, orthopedic, and OB/GYN service lines.

- Assisted surgeons by anticipating procedural needs,

selecting appropriate instruments, and maintaining sterile field integrity.

• Performed surgical counts with zero discrepancies across more than 900 cases.

• Supported laparoscopic and robotic procedures, including equipment setup and troubleshooting.

• Collaborated with circulating nurses, anesthesia teams, and surgeons to ensure efficient workflow and safe patient care.

New graduates should list clinical rotations using the same structure, including procedure types and specialties.

7. Specialty Experience Section (Optional)

Provide a concise list of specialties you are comfortable scrubbing, such as general surgery, orthopedics, OB/GYN, ENT, plastics, urology, or laparoscopic surgery. Highlight robotics or cardiothoracic experience if applicable.

8. Technical Skills and Equipment Proficiency

Include sterilization systems, documentation platforms, laparoscopic towers, robotic systems, surgical scopes, orthopedic power tools, or other specialty equipment you routinely use.

9. Professional and Interpersonal Skills

Include communication, adaptability to surgeon preferences, situational awareness, stress management, teamwork, and time management. Interpersonal performance is a major factor in operating room success.

Part III: Tailoring Your Résumé for Operating Room Hiring Managers

Lead with specialties, quantify experience whenever possible, use terminology familiar to surgical services such as sterile field, counts, preference cards, and turnover, and maintain a clean bullet-point format. Avoid long narrative blocks; clarity and readability are critical.

Part IV: What Hiring Managers Notice Immediately

Hiring managers focus on certification status, specialty experience, reliability under pressure, communication professionalism, and familiarity with operating room workflow. They do not need unrelated job history or lengthy non-clinical descriptions.

Part V: Sample High-Impact Bullet Points

• Supported more than 1,000 surgical procedures with full compliance to sterile technique standards and AORN (gl) guidelines.

• Anticipated surgeon needs by mastering preference cards and procedural sequencing across multiple specialties.

• Reduced room turnover time by improving supply readiness and workflow coordination.

• Assisted with robotic and laparoscopic procedures, including docking preparation and equipment troubleshooting.

• Collaborated with interdisciplinary teams to ensure safe patient positioning, specimen handling, and accurate documentation.

Final Words to Future Surgical Technologists

Your résumé speaks for you before you ever enter the operating room. Keep it precise, structured, and clear. When written well, it communicates that you understand sterile discipline, surgical workflow, patient safety, and team collaboration—and that you are ready to contribute from day one.

Chapter 18
Interview Preparation for Surgical Technologist

Interview Prep for Surgical Technologists

How to Show Confidence, Technical Skill, and OR Readiness in Every Interview

The operating room is one of the most rhythm-dependent, trust-dependent, and detail-dependent environments in healthcare. Surgical Technologists are not hired on résumé alone; they are hired on poise, precision, and the unspoken question every surgeon and OR leader asks: *Can I trust this person with my sterile field and with my patient?* This chapter provides a clear framework for entering every interview with confidence, preparation, and the language operating room leaders expect to hear.

Part I: What OR Leaders Are Really Evaluating

A Surgical Services Manager or OR Director evaluates more than technical skill. They are assessing sterile technique mastery, the ability to anticipate surgeon needs, composure under pressure, competency across service lines, communication with circulating nurses and anesthesia teams, team reliability, and commitment to patient safety. They are not hiring your résumé alone; they are hiring your situational awareness.

Part II: The Six Categories of Surgical Technologist Interview Questions

1. Technical and Sterile Technique Questions

These questions test foundational operating room practice. Common examples include: “Walk me through how you set up your sterile field,” “How do you handle a contaminated instrument during a procedure?” “Describe the steps for performing a surgical count,” and “How do you ensure sterility when passing instruments?” Interviewers listen for confidence, clarity, and consistent sterile protocol.

2. Surgical Sequence and Anticipation Questions

These questions assess whether you think ahead during procedures. Examples include: “How do you prepare for a surgeon you have never worked with?” “How do you anticipate needs during laparoscopic procedures?” and “What signs tell you a surgeon is moving to the next step?” Candidates should reference real case experiences whenever possible.

3. Case-Based Scenario Questions

These simulate real operating room situations. Examples include: “What would you do if a count were incorrect?” “How do you manage tension when a surgeon becomes frustrated?” “Describe a time you recognized a problem early,” or “Tell me about a complication you witnessed and how the team responded." Interviewers evaluate calm reasoning, prioritization, escalation awareness, and patient-first thinking.

4. Service Line Experience Questions

Hiring leaders need to understand where you can function confidently. Expect questions such as: "Which specialties are you strongest in?" "Which procedures do you scrub most frequently?" "Do you have robotics experience?" or "What is your comfort level with orthopedic power tools or endoscopic towers?" Honest, specific answers build trust.

5. Communication and Team Dynamics Questions

Because operating rooms function under pressure, communication style matters. Examples include: "How do you communicate with a new surgeon?" "How do you handle conflicting directions?" "Describe your relationship with circulating nurses," or "What does effective teamwork look like in the OR?" Leaders seek calm, respectful, direct communicators who will speak up if safety is compromised.

6. Professionalism and Reliability Questions

These questions address dependability. Examples include: "Describe your punctuality and attendance," "How do you handle high-volume days?" "What motivates you in the OR?" and "Why do you want to work with our team?" Prepare concise examples that demonstrate consistency and reliability.

Part III: Preparing Before the Interview

1. Know Your Service Lines

Review your case types, approximate case numbers, specialty strengths, and experience with robotics, scopes, or power tools so you can discuss them confidently.

2. Review Sterile Technique Fundamentals

Be ready to describe how you open sterile supplies, gown and glove, identify contamination, and correct contamination calmly. Clear explanations signal readiness.

3. Prepare Signature Case Stories

Develop three to five brief examples that demonstrate anticipation, communication, technical ability, calm decision-making, and patient-safety awareness. Structure responses using Situation → Action → Outcome.

4. Practice Walking Through a Case

Interviewers often ask candidates to describe how they prepare for a procedure, anticipate surgical steps, conduct counts, and manage turnover. Choose one familiar case—such as laparoscopic cholecystectomy, cesarean section, open reduction internal fixation (ORIF) (gl), hernia repair, or hysteroscopy—and practice explaining the full workflow.

Part IV: What to Expect on Interview Day

Many Surgical Technologist interviews include an operating room walk-through. Interviewers observe how comfortable you appear in the environment, how you discuss equipment, and whether you understand layout, workflow, and sterile boundaries. You may also be asked real-time situational questions such as identifying setup issues, positioning considerations, or missing instruments from a Mayo setup.

Part V: Questions You Should Ask the Employer

Strong candidates ask thoughtful questions such as:

- Which service lines currently need the most coverage?
- How many operating rooms will I rotate through?
- What is the orientation structure for new Surgical Technologists?
- Which specialties or surgeons will I work with most often?
- What major systems are used here (robotics, laparoscopic platforms, sterilization equipment)?

Questions focused on workflow and expectations demonstrate professional maturity.

Part VI: Demonstrating OR-Level Professionalism

Arrive early, dress professionally, communicate calmly, and emphasize patient safety, accuracy, teamwork, reliability, and surgeon support. The operating room is a professional culture; interviews assess whether you will integrate smoothly into that environment.

Final Words to Future Surgical Technologists

A strong Surgical Technologist is a technician, communicator, protector of the sterile field, and advocate for patient safety. In the interview, your goal is to show calm decision-making, technical readiness, collaborative mindset, and respect for the rhythm of the operating room. Confidence and clarity signal that you are ready to contribute from day one.

Chapter 19

Behavioral Interviewing for Surgical Technologist

Healthcare organizations do not hire solely on credentials, certifications, or technical checklists. They hire based on how professionals actually behave when real patients, real pressure, and real uncertainty are present. Behavioral interviewing is designed to reveal this difference. Instead of asking what you *would* do, behavioral interview questions ask what you *have done*. Past behavior is considered one of the strongest predictors of future performance, especially in environments like the operating room where judgment, communication, and composure directly affect patient safety.

In surgical services, hiring leaders are not simply evaluating whether you understand sterile technique or instrument handling. They are trying to determine how you think under pressure, how you communicate when stress rises, how you respond when something goes wrong, and whether you consistently prioritize patient safety over convenience or speed. Behavioral questions allow them to see evidence of these qualities through real experiences rather than hypothetical answers.

This approach is especially important in the operating room because the OR is a trust-dependent environment. Surgeons, nurses, anesthesia professionals, and surgical technologists function as an interdependent team. A single lapse in communication, hesitation during a critical moment, or failure to speak up when sterility is compromised can have serious consequences. Behavioral interviewing helps leaders identify candidates who demonstrate accountability, teamwork, calm decision-making, and the ability to act decisively when patient safety is at stake.

Fortunately, behavioral interviewing is highly learnable. Candidates who understand the structure behind these questions can respond clearly, confidently, and consistently. One of the most effective frameworks for answering behavioral questions is the **EAR™ Method**:

E — Event

A — Action

R — Result

This simple structure helps transform a scattered story into a focused professional example that interviewers can easily follow.

Event refers to the situation or context. Briefly describe what was happening. Keep this portion concise—just enough information to help the interviewer understand the environment and stakes involved. For example, you might describe an emergency case, a challenging turnover day, a complex surgical procedure, or a moment when sterility was at risk.

Action explains what *you* specifically did. This is the most important part of the answer. Hiring leaders want to understand your decision-making, your communication style, and how you contributed to the team. Focus on the behaviors that demonstrate professionalism, safety awareness, anticipation, teamwork, and accountability.

Result describes what happened because of those actions. Whenever possible, connect the outcome to patient safety, improved efficiency, better teamwork, or prevention of an error. Even when discussing a mistake, the "result" should highlight what was learned and how your practice improved afterward.

A strong EAR™ response might sound like this:

- **Event:** "During a laparoscopic procedure, I noticed a discrepancy between the requested instrument and the one placed on the field."
- **Action:** "I paused briefly to confirm the instrument size with the surgeon before passing it and retrieved the correct instrument immediately."
- **Result:** "The correction prevented a delay in the procedure and reinforced the importance of double-checking instruments before use."

Notice how the example stays focused, concise, and centered on safety and teamwork. Interviewers are not looking for dramatic storytelling; they are looking for clarity, ownership, and evidence of professional judgment.

Behavioral interviewing also serves another purpose: it allows organizations to assess reliability and cultural fit. Healthcare leaders want to know whether you arrive prepared, communicate respectfully, adapt to different surgeon styles, support teammates during stressful moments, and maintain professionalism even when cases become difficult. The way you describe your past experiences often reveals these qualities more clearly than any résumé bullet point.

Preparing for behavioral interviews means thinking ahead about real moments from your clinical training, rotations, or professional experience. Identify situations that demonstrate calmness under pressure, advocacy for patient safety, adaptability, teamwork, learning a new skill quickly, handling feedback constructively, or improving workflow efficiency. When you rehearse these experiences using the EAR™ framework, your answers become organized, confident, and easy for interviewers to evaluate.

Ultimately, behavioral interviewing is not designed to "trap" candidates. It exists because healthcare environments require professionals who can consistently translate knowledge into safe action. By understanding why these questions are asked and using the EAR™ Method to structure your responses, you can walk into any Surgical Technologist interview prepared to show not only what you know—but how you perform when it matters most.

Behavioral Interviewing Questions

Surgeons evaluate your hands. Operating room leaders evaluate your teamwork. Organizations evaluate your reliability. Behavioral interviewing is where these elements meet. These questions are not designed to test technical memorization; they are intended to reveal how you respond to pressure, conflict, fatigue, and real clinical responsibility. Strong answers show identity, judgment, and professionalism in action.

1. "Tell me about a time you had to stay calm during an emergency."

Sample response: During an emergency trauma case involving severe internal bleeding, I focused on maintaining steady breathing and immediately followed my mental setup checklist. I anticipated the surgeon's needs, opened additional trays, and prepared vascular clamps in advance. Remaining calm allowed the team to function cohesively and reinforced the importance of emotional steadiness during crisis situations.

2. "Describe a time you disagreed with a surgeon or coworker."

Sample response: During a laparoscopic case, I noticed a potential break in sterile positioning as equipment was being adjusted. I calmly said, "Let me assist so we maintain the sterile field," and repositioned the equipment appropriately. After the case, I briefly explained the situation to ensure shared understanding. The interaction reinforced that respectful communication protects patient safety.

3. "Tell me about a mistake you made and how you handled it."

Sample response: Early in my training, I opened a package that was later identified as non-sterile. I immediately notified the team, removed the item, and replaced it before the procedure continued. The experience reinforced that immediate transparency is essential to maintaining patient safety.

4. "Describe a time you adapted to a surgeon's unique style."

Sample response: When working with a surgeon who preferred minimal verbal communication, I studied his case sequence and instrument preferences in advance. By anticipating needs more precisely, our workflow became smoother, and the surgeon later commented on the improved efficiency of the case.

5. "Give an example of how you manage long, physically demanding cases."

Sample response: During extended spine procedures lasting several hours, I maintain endurance by adjusting posture, staying mentally engaged in the case sequence, and preparing instruments in advance so the pace remains controlled through closure.

6. "Tell me about a time you prevented an error."

Sample response: During a laparoscopic case, I noticed that an instrument prepared for use did not match the requested size. I clarified the selection before it was passed, preventing a potential delay and reinforcing the importance of verification.

7. "Describe a time you supported a struggling teammate."

Sample response: When a new team member felt overwhelmed during a busy turnover period, I assisted with setup and calmly walked through the instrument sequence.

Supporting colleagues strengthens team performance and improves overall workflow.

8. "Give an example of how you handled conflict in the OR."

Sample response: During a high-stress case, communication tension arose between team members. I focused on maintaining clear task prioritization and calmly redirected attention to the next surgical step, which helped stabilize the environment until the procedure concluded.

9. "Tell me about a time you had to learn a new skill quickly."

Sample response: When a new robotic platform was introduced, I reviewed instructional materials, practiced equipment setup before scheduled cases, and worked with vendor educators to ensure I could support procedures confidently once the system went live.

10. "Describe a time you advocated for patient safety."

Sample response: Before a procedure, I noticed compromised packaging on an implant. I requested a replacement immediately, ensuring sterility standards were maintained even though it delayed the start slightly.

11. "Tell me about a time you handled turnover pressure."

Sample response: During a series of rapid orthopedic cases, I standardized my instrument layout and pre-labeled sutures between procedures, helping the team maintain efficient turnover times without compromising preparation quality.

12. "Give an example of how you handled feedback."

Sample response: After receiving feedback about instrument passing technique, I practiced the preferred positioning until it became consistent. Feedback allows refinement of technique and strengthens teamwork.

13. "Tell me about a time communication prevented a problem."

Sample response: During a laparoscopic procedure, I observed irregular insufflation pressure readings and immediately notified the team. Equipment connections were corrected quickly, preventing case delay.

14. "Describe a situation where you had to manage multiple priorities."

Sample response: During a complex case requiring multiple instrument sequences, I prioritized tasks based on procedural steps, ensuring that safety-critical items were always prepared before efficiency-related tasks.

15. "Tell me about a time you improved efficiency."

Sample response: I created a standardized checklist for frequently used trays within our service line, which reduced retrieval time and improved consistency between cases.

16. "Describe how you handled emotional stress after a difficult case."

Sample response: After a particularly challenging case, I spoke briefly with colleagues and took time to decompress before returning to the schedule, recognizing the importance of maintaining emotional resilience.

17. "Tell me about a time you worked with a challenging personality."

Sample response: By observing communication preferences and adjusting my interaction style, I was able to develop a more productive working relationship, improving case flow over time.

18. "Describe a time you took initiative without being asked."

Sample response: During a case with unexpected blood loss, I prepared additional suction equipment and supplies in advance, allowing the team to respond quickly as the situation evolved.

19. "Tell me about a time you earned a surgeon's trust."

Sample response: By consistently preparing instruments accurately and anticipating procedural steps over multiple cases, I demonstrated reliability that strengthened working trust.

20. "Describe a time you turned a difficult situation into a positive outcome."

Sample response: After an equipment delay, I reorganized the setup and prepared additional supplies so the case could proceed efficiently once the issue was resolved, helping the team recover lost time.

Chapter 20

Introduction to the SCRUBfits™

Identity Mirrors Inside the Surgical Technologist Role

Every operating room runs on teamwork, precision, and rhythm, but not every Surgical Technologist experiences that rhythm the same way. Some thrive on pace. Some thrive on structure. Others love the equipment, the systems, or the high-pressure urgency that certain cases bring. The **SCRUB*fits*™** are not personality labels; they are alignment mirrors designed to help you notice which parts of the OR environment energize you and which parts quietly drain you. As you read this spotlight, pay attention to what feels familiar. That recognition often tells you more than any checklist ever could.

Sergi Tekno is the Rhythm Builder. Sergi thrives in flow. Instrument sequencing, preference cards, surgeon patterns, and smooth turnovers create a deep sense of professional satisfaction. When the case runs cleanly and the team moves almost without speaking, Sergi feels fully in the zone. Surgical Technologists who recognize themselves here usually enjoy repetition mastery, efficiency, and the quiet pride of making complex procedures feel seamless. They tend to value predictability inside the chaos, preparation over improvisation, and the kind of competence that shows up as calm. For them, the operating room becomes most satisfying when the day has a steady tempo, the setup is exact, the room is disciplined, and the work feels like choreography: intentional, practiced, and precise.

You may recognize yourself strongly in Sergi's spotlight, or you may simply notice moments of connection. Either is useful. Alignment is rarely a single label; it is a pattern that becomes clearer over time. As you move through this book, notice which operating-room environments, specialties, and workflow styles consistently bring out your best performance and your most sustainable energy. That awareness is one of the most valuable career signals you can develop early.

Chapter 21
Day In The Life

Welcome to Your 15 Days in the Life

Real Moments. Real Rhythm. Real Life in the OR.

Before you step behind the double doors and into the pressure, pace, and precision of the operating room, I want you to understand something important:

There is no such thing as a "typical day" for a Surgical Technologist.

Some days are smooth, structured, and satisfyingly predictable.

Some days are chaotic and adrenaline-charged.

Some days will test your stamina.

Others will remind you why you chose this path in the first place.

These 15 Day-In-The-Life vignettes are designed to show you the full spectrum — the good, the gritty, the meaningful, the unforgettable, and the quietly heroic moments that shape the life of a Surgical Technologist.

You'll see:

- The early mornings where the OR hums before sunrise
- The sudden emergencies that change everything
- The delicate cases that require absolute silence
- The long, complex procedures that demand endurance
- The teamwork that holds the entire room together
- The quiet victories no patient ever sees

Each vignette drops you right into the room — gowning, gloving, counting, passing instruments, anticipating needs, protecting the sterile field, and supporting the surgeon through every critical moment.

Some of these days will make you nod and say, "Yes — this is exactly what it feels like."

Some will make you think, "I hope I get to do that one day."

And some will make you pause and think about alignment — about the pace, the environment, the specialties, and the teams where *you* will thrive.

That's the purpose of these vignettes:

To let you experience the OR without stepping into it.

To show you what's possible.

To help you feel the rhythm before you ever touch a Mayo stand.

So take a deep breath. Tie your mask. Adjust your eye shield.

The lights are bright.

The room is chilled.

The sterile field is ready.

And you're about to step into 15 real, lived-in windows into the world of Surgical Technology.

Welcome to the OR.

Let's begin.

Chapter 22
Day in The Life — Level 1 Trauma Center

Day in the Life Level I Trauma Center

15:05 — Your call shift starts later, but your body starts preparing early. At home, your French Bulldog, Mochi, follows you from room to room with that stubborn little shadow energy, as if your bag is the reason you're leaving—not the job. You scratch behind his ears while you do the mental inventory you always do before trauma call (gl): phone charged, snacks packed, badge where it should be, and a brain that's trying not to sprint ahead of the night.

15:30 — Your day starts when most people are winding theirs down. While friends are texting about dinner plans and streaming shows, you're looking at the calendar and seeing one word that changes everything: call. Overnight trauma call (gl) at a Level I trauma center (gl) is not the same as a regular shift. You are not just planning for a busy night; you are preparing for the possibility of anything. You eat an early, heavier meal than usual—something with protein and carbs—because you know there may be long stretches where you cannot leave the OR (gl) long enough to grab more than a sip of water.

16:15 — You pack your bag differently on call days. Extra snacks, a phone charger, a sweatshirt for the cold ORs, and maybe a small notebook where you sometimes jot down things you want to remember or process later. You check your call start and end times again: 19:00 to 07:00. Officially twelve hours, but you know that turning your brain off at 07:01 is not realistic. You glance at your phone, see the latest group chat string of memes, and type a quick message: "On trauma call tonight. Text me something dumb at 02:00." You mean it. Sometimes a ridiculous emoji is the perfect anchor in the middle of chaos.

17:00 — Before you leave, you try to bank a little rest. You darken your room, silence most notifications, and set a gentle alarm. You are not really asleep, but you let your body sink into stillness. You know from experience that the quality of your early-night calls—how calm your hands feel, how steady your focus stays—depends partly on this half-nap. You are not tired yet, but you will be. You are making a down payment on the effort to come.

18:20 — The sky is in that in-between color when you pull into the hospital parking lot, not fully dark but clearly moving that way. Walking toward the entrance, you feel the difference between this and a day shift. Fewer people, less chatter, more echo in the halls. You badge in, change into scrubs (gl), and clip your call pager (gl) to your waistband. In the core, the board shows the evening elective cases finishing up: a laparoscopic (gl) case in OR 2, a spine case in OR 5, a C-section (gl) on the labor and delivery board. Your name is listed under "Trauma OR," with a note: "On call 19:00-07:00."

18:45 — You check with the charge nurse and the trauma coordinator. "Nothing inbound right now," they say, "but EMS (gl) has already had a busy evening." You walk to the designated trauma OR to make sure it is ready. Trauma feels like an exam you cannot study for, but you can at least sharpen your pencils. You check that you have a basic set-up: trauma laparotomy (gl) tray, vascular instruments, large retractors, extra suction (gl), rapid infuser (gl) connection ready, cell saver (gl) machine parked and plugged in. You confirm that blood products are easily accessible and that the massive transfusion protocol (gl) chart is visible on the wall.

You do not know what kind of case will hit your door, but you know the themes: bleeding, broken, unstable. The trauma bay (gl) downstairs does the first sorting; you are the second line when the decision is made that someone needs the OR now.

19:10 — The pager goes off for the first time: a long-tone vibration that still makes your stomach tighten, even though you have heard it countless times. "Trauma activation. ETA 10 minutes. MVC (gl), rollover, multiple patients." You listen to the overhead announcement as you head toward the trauma bay: "Trauma team to the emergency department."

19:20 — In the trauma bay, the world narrows to bright lights, fast voices, and organized movement. EMS wheels in a patient in a cervical collar (gl), clothes cut away, dried blood on their face. You stand slightly back, out of the way of the primary survey, but close enough to hear the report. You listen for certain words: "unstable," "positive FAST (gl)," "taken directly to CT (gl)," "going to the OR now." Sometimes you can feel the decision forming before anyone says it out loud—the tilt in the room, the shift from assessment to action.

19:35 — Back in the trauma OR, you move fast but not frantic. You open the emergency laparotomy set, more retractors, vascular clamps (gl), aortic cross-clamp (gl), and extra suction tubing. You build the table like you're building an answer key: what the surgeon will need first, what they'll need when things get ugly, what they'll need if the bleeding won't stop. The surgeon does a rapid timeout (gl), confirming identity and procedure, and then the room tightens into that familiar, controlled urgency.

20:00 — Time becomes strange once the abdomen is open. You pass suction tips, long clamps, sponges. The surgeon's voice is calm but clipped, the kind of calm that doesn't waste air. Anesthesia calls out numbers that matter more than conversation: blood pressure dropping, heart rate climbing, unit counts climbing with it. The rapid infuser hums like a machine that doesn't care how late it is. The cell saver cycles, spinning blood back toward usefulness. Your job is to keep the field clean, the instruments ready, and your own hands steady even when your brain wants to match the room's speed.

You learn to read the surgeon's body language in trauma: the way their shoulders set when they find the source, the half-second pause when they don't. You anticipate without guessing. You pass without rushing. You count without missing. In the middle of it, you are not thinking about how loud the monitors are. You are thinking about the next request before it becomes a request.

00:20 — The pager vibrates again. This time the message is shorter and sharper: "Trauma alert. GSW (gl) to abdomen. ETA

5 minutes." That sentence lands in the room like a dropped tray—everyone hears it, even if they pretend they don't. You glance at the clock and feel the night split into a before and after. You are already moving, already stripping down what you can, already preparing for the next set-up while the current one is still trying to end.

00:40 – You help pack the abdomen with laparotomy sponges (gl) and assist with suction while the surgeon makes the fastest safe decisions they can. The goal is survival first, perfection later. When the patient finally leaves the room, the space they occupied feels briefly haunted—blood cleaned, drapes gone, instruments sent away—but the pressure lingers. You reset your table like a reflex, because the next patient will not wait for you to feel ready.

02:10 – When this case ends, the patient goes to the intensive care unit (gl) with drains, lines, and a chart full of orders. You watch the bed roll out and feel the strange mixture that comes with trauma call: relief that they're alive, uncertainty about what "alive" will look like tomorrow, and the quiet knowledge that your pager can still go off again before the night is done.

SCRUB*fits*™ Reflection – Sergi Tekno

"If you felt yourself relax during the moments when the room ran smoothly – when the setup was exact, the surgeon's rhythm was familiar, and the team seemed to communicate without words – that is an alignment signal. Many Surgical Technologists thrive when preparation turns into flow, and competence feels like calm."

Chapter 23

Day In The Life — Outpatient Surgery Center

Day in the Life Outpatient Surgery Center

04:50 — Your alarm goes off in the dark, but this early start feels different from trauma call. Outpatient surgery center days promise something closer to predictability: a packed schedule of shorter cases with a strong chance of being home for dinner. You lie there for a second, thinking about the list you checked last night: hernia repairs, laparoscopic (gl) gallbladders, small orthopedic scopes, and a couple of plastics cases.

05:45 — The parking lot at the surgery center feels different from the big hospital. Smaller building, fewer floors, one main entrance. You park close, badge in, and head straight to the locker room. Changing into scrubs feels like shrugging into a slightly different identity. You walk into the core, where the hall is lined with smaller operating rooms, each door labeled.

06:00 — You check the board and see your name assigned to OR 2 all day. Inside the room, you begin waking the space up

—checking suction and the electrocautery unit before opening the laparoscopic trays: trocars (gl), camera system, insufflator (gl), clamps, scissors, and forceps. Sutures are lined up along with dressings and local anesthetic (gl).

06:25 — You step into pre-op to introduce yourself to the first patient and explain your role protecting the sterile field once surgery begins. Even in shorter outpatient cases, that reassurance matters.

06:45 — Anesthesia places an airway device—often an LMA (gl)—and confirms stable vitals. Soon you are passing the first instruments: Veress needle (gl), trocar, camera. When the gallbladder anatomy appears on the screen, you anticipate the next step and prepare the clip applier (gl).

08:05 — The first case ends, and the patient heads to PACU. You begin turnover, wiping surfaces, sending instruments to sterile processing, and preparing the next case while maintaining strict infection-prevention standards.

10:30 — Mid-morning brings the scope run: three arthroscopic (gl) knee cases in a row. Towers, cameras, and the fluid pump (gl) are checked again as instruments move through surgical portals (gl) during each procedure.

12:20 — Afternoon plastics cases include a blepharoplasty (gl). The trays contain finer instruments, and your movements become more deliberate, almost slower, even though the schedule remains tight.

15:45 — As the final case closes, the pace finally loosens. Outpatient surgery days carry a different kind of fatigue—not the adrenaline drain of trauma, but the steady burn of repetition, precision, and speed. When you change out of scrubs and step into the daylight, there is a small but meaningful satisfaction in knowing that, barring add-ons, your evening will belong to you.

Chapter 24

Day In The Life — Pediatrics ENT

Day in the Life Pediatric Hospital

05:30 — Your alarm feels a little gentler this morning, partly because you went to bed knowing exactly what kind of day you were walking into. Today you are at the children's hospital, assigned to the ENT (ear, nose, and throat) (gl) service. Instead of hips, knees, or trauma, your cases will be tonsillectomies (gl), adenoidectomies (gl), and ear tube placements (tympanostomy tubes) (gl) on kids who are still learning to tie their shoes.

06:10 — You badge in, change into scrubs, and check the OR board. First up: a six-year-old with enlarged tonsils. Pediatric days carry a different emotional tone—more parents at the bedside, more reassurance needed, and a quiet understanding that small procedures can feel very big to small patients.

06:30 — In OR 3, you prepare the room and open ENT trays: small retractors, tonsil snares (gl), mouth gags (gl), and pediatric suction tips. For ear tube cases, you set aside speculums (gl) and microinstruments (gl), keeping the table organized for the rapid pace these procedures often require.

06:50 — In pre-op, you meet the first patient and their parent. A child life specialist (gl) kneels next to the stretcher, using distraction tools and playful conversation to lower anxiety. You introduce yourself and explain your role, knowing the parent is listening just as closely as the child.

07:15 — After the child is asleep, anesthesia secures the airway using an endotracheal tube (gl). The surgeon begins the tonsillectomy, and you pass instruments steadily, keeping suction clear as tissue is removed. When bleeding is controlled and hemostasis (gl) is achieved, the procedure concludes quickly compared to many adult surgeries.

08:05 — The child is extubated (gl) and transported to recovery. You complete counts and begin turnover, resetting the room for the next patient while maintaining the steady rhythm of pediatric surgery days.

12:30 — The afternoon includes a more complex airway case involving obstructive sleep apnea (gl), requiring specialized instruments and slower, more deliberate pacing. Even routine pediatric surgeries demand careful positioning and constant awareness of smaller anatomical structures.

15:45 — Standing in the OR afterward, you notice the pediatric-size equipment laid out across the back table—the tiny cuffs, delicate instruments, and scaled-down supplies that quietly remind you how different children's surgery is from adult cases. Pediatric days often end earlier than trauma or inpatient schedules, but the emotional energy is unique: a mix of technical focus, family reassurance, and the quiet satisfaction of seeing young patients wake up safely.

SCRUB*fits*™ Reflection — Sergi Tekno

"Notice whether you enjoy repetition mastery. In the OR, doing the same procedure many times is not boredom for the right person — it is refinement. If improving efficiency, sequencing, and anticipation feels satisfying to you, this role can become deeply rewarding over time."

Chapter 25
Day In The Life — Labor and Delivery

Day in the Life Labor and Delivery OR

05:15 — Your alarm goes off and for a second you forget which board you're on. Then you remember: you are assigned to the Labor and Delivery (L&D) ORs today, a world where surgery and childbirth collide. You eat breakfast with that in mind, choosing something steady and filling. Today's list includes scheduled C-sections (cesarean deliveries) for breech (gl) babies and repeat moms who have had them before, but you also know the truth: L&D days rarely stick to the script. Somewhere between the printed schedule and reality, emergencies can and do appear.

05:50 — The hospital looks almost sleepy from the outside, but as you badge in and take the elevator to the L&D floor, you feel a different kind of energy. Labor rooms are already occupied; monitors glow with fetal heart rate (gl) tracings and contraction patterns. You change into scrubs, pull on dedicated L&D shoe covers, and clip your badge. At the nurses' station, the charge nurse points you toward the small cluster of ORs off the main labor hallway. The dry-erase board lists two scheduled C-sections this morning and space for STAT (urgent) cases that might appear without warning.

06:10 — In the first L&D OR, you begin your setup, opening the C-section trays and arranging scalpel, clamps, scissors, forceps, retractors, needle holders, and suture (gl) materials. You prepare the newborn warmer with blankets and caps, aware that this side of the room carries its own gravity. Medications used for uterine contraction and local anesthetic supplies are checked, and you confirm blood products are available if needed.

06:35 — In pre-op, you meet your first patient and introduce yourself as part of the OR team who will assist during the birth. A mix of excitement and anxiety is visible on the patient's face, mirrored by the partner sitting beside her. The anesthesiologist explains the spinal anesthesia plan while nurses prepare final paperwork and monitoring.

07:05 — Back in the OR, draping begins once anesthesia confirms the block is effective. A sterile drape separates the surgical field from the patient's head, where the support person sits holding her hand. You focus on the lower field, organizing instruments and anticipating the surgeon's next request.

07:20 — The incision begins. You pass instruments steadily as the surgeon moves through tissue layers, including the fascia (gl), toward the uterus. Moments later, the pace shifts slightly as delivery approaches. With assistance, the baby is delivered, the cord is clamped and cut, and the newborn is transferred to the waiting neonatal team.

07:31 — The baby's first cry fills the room. While family members meet their newborn, the surgical team continues working. After the placenta (gl) is delivered, uterine repair begins and closure proceeds layer by layer, with careful counts of sponges, needles, and instruments maintained throughout.

09:30 — A second scheduled C-section follows with a similar technical process but a completely different family story. Scar tissue from prior surgery requires slower dissection, yet the delivery is smooth and the newborn arrives healthy. Even when procedures feel routine, each birth carries a unique emotional landscape.

11:10 — Mid-morning, the board changes: "Add-on STAT C-section - fetal distress (gl)." The atmosphere tightens. You prepare the second OR rapidly—opening trays, confirming neonatal warmer readiness, and setting out additional hemorrhage (gl) supplies. This is the unpredictable side of L&D surgery.

11:35 — The patient arrives quickly, and anesthesia induces anesthesia while the surgical team prepares. Once the incision begins, the pace is faster than in scheduled cases. Instruments move rapidly but methodically as the team works to deliver the baby as efficiently and safely as possible. After a tense moment, the newborn cries, releasing a wave of relief across the room.

13:30 — A late lunch offers a short pause while the emotional intensity of the morning settles. Conversations in the break room alternate between clinical discussion and light humor—the balance many teams rely on to decompress.

14:10 — The afternoon is quieter: smaller procedures, restocking supplies, and assisting where needed. You check trays, replenish sutures, and ensure medications such as uterotonics (gl) are ready for the evening shift.

17:05 — After giving report to the incoming team, you change back into your clothes and leave the unit. Photos of newborns line the hallway, quiet reminders of the families whose stories briefly intersected with yours today.

21:15 — In bed that night, the day plays back in fragments: a first cry, a moment of urgency, a team moving together in practiced rhythm. Some people find the emotional intensity of L&D overwhelming; others find meaning in standing at the intersection of surgery and the beginning of life. Days like this help you understand where you might fall on that spectrum.

Chapter 26

Day In The Life — Open Heart Surgery

Day in the Life Cardiac OR

04:30 — The alarm goes off in the kind of dark that feels deeper than usual. Cardiac OR days start early, and they demand a different kind of readiness. You lie still for a moment, feeling the weight of what is ahead. Open-heart surgery is not just another case type; it is a full-body, full-brain commitment from everyone in the room. You roll out of bed, feet hitting the floor with a small thud, and head to the kitchen. Breakfast is not optional today. You choose something solid—eggs, toast, maybe oatmeal—and drink water even though you are not really thirsty yet. You know how hot and dry those lights can feel four hours into a case.

05:10 — On your phone, you open the hospital schedule. Your name is next to "Cardiac OR 1," with a first case listed as "CABG x3" (coronary artery bypass graft) (gl). Under it, there is a valve replacement and a "possible add-on" slot that could turn into anything—perhaps an aortic dissection (gl). You mentally run through what you know about today's surgeon: fast but meticulous, particular about instruments, quiet when focused. You pack snacks, your water bottle, and a sweatshirt you can throw on if you get chilled during a long bypass run.

05:45 — The hospital is still sleepy when you walk in, but the cardiac wing never really feels off-duty. In the cardiac area, you see perfusionists (gl) checking the heart-lung machine (gl), anesthesia setting up advanced monitors, and another tech preparing a back table in the next room. The board confirms your assignment: CABG followed by aortic valve replacement.

06:00 — Inside the room, preparation begins: suction tested, cautery checked, and the cell saver (gl) ready. You open cardiac trays—sternotomy (gl) instruments, long vascular clamps (gl), delicate forceps, and sternal saw (gl) components—arranging sutures by size and type for rapid access.

06:30 — In pre-op, you meet the patient and introduce yourself as part of the surgical team. Their family sits nearby asking quiet questions about timing and recovery. You answer what you can and reassure them that the team will remain focused on the patient throughout the procedure.

06:50 — Back in the room, anesthesia places invasive monitoring lines including an arterial line (gl), central venous catheter (gl), and sometimes a pulmonary artery catheter (gl). Draping is completed carefully, and bypass cannulation (gl) instruments are arranged within reach.

07:20 — The first incision is made. After the sternum is opened and the mediastinum (gl) exposed, you assist as the surgeon prepares for bypass. Cannulas (gl) are placed into the aorta (gl) and right atrium (gl), connecting circulation to the heart-lung machine. Once cardioplegia (gl) solution is delivered, the heart temporarily stops, allowing the surgeon to perform delicate coronary artery (gl) grafting work.

10:15 — A brief bleeding issue requires additional sutures and suction, but the situation stabilizes quickly. As the team prepares to come off bypass, the heart resumes beating and circulation transitions back to the patient.

11:30 — Chest tubes (gl) are placed, and the sternum is secured with sternal wires (gl) before closure. Final counts are verified carefully before the patient is transferred to the ICU.

13:00 — The second case begins: valve replacement surgery. You pass valve sizers (gl), prosthetic valves (gl), and sutures prepared with pledgets (gl), maintaining the same careful rhythm that defines cardiac cases.

17:30 — After final turnover and supply restocking, you give a handoff to the evening team. Cardiac days are long, demanding, and intensely focused, but they carry a quiet sense of accomplishment when the room finally settles.

18:40 — At home, the day plays back in fragments—the stillness of the arrested heart, the steady return of rhythm, and the teamwork required to make each step possible. Cardiac OR work is not for everyone, but for those drawn to precision under pressure, it can feel deeply meaningful.

SCRUB*fits*™ Reflection — Sergi Tekno

"Preference cards and surgeon patterns can feel either grounding or frustrating. If you like learning the details that

keep a case running cleanly — which instruments come next, how a surgeon sets up, what reduces delays — you may be naturally aligned with the rhythm-building side of surgical technology."

Chapter 27

Day In The Life — Neurology

Day in the Life Neuro OR

05:10 — Your alarm cuts through the quiet while the apartment is still dark. Your border collie, Dash, lifts his head from the foot of the bed, ears alert even at this early hour, then settles back down when he realizes you are the one getting up. In the kitchen, you prepare a deliberate breakfast—eggs, toast, and fruit—because neuro cases demand long stretches of concentration and there is no convenient moment to step away once a procedure begins. While coffee brews, you glance at the day's assignment message: Neuro OR 2. Spine and brain cases. High-precision work, long hours, and a level of focus that leaves little room for distraction.

05:45 — Coffee in hand, you open the hospital schedule on your phone. First case: lumbar laminectomy and fusion (gl) for a patient with severe back and leg pain. Second case: craniotomy (gl) for tumor resection. A third block reads "TBD," which in a neuro service can quickly become an emergency aneurysm (gl) or trauma add-on. You pack snacks, water, and a hoodie—neuro rooms often run cold to support equipment performance and infection control.

06:20 — The walk from the parking garage feels routine, but mentally you are already building the room setup. After changing into scrubs, you review the board again: neuro monitoring (gl) scheduled, anesthesia assignments confirmed, surgeon listed. You remember this surgeon prefers a precise instrument layout and microscope positioning. Not a problem —predictability helps the case flow.

06:35 — Neuro OR 2 is quiet as you begin opening spine trays: retractors, rongeurs (gl), curettes (gl), drills, and fusion implants. The surgical microscope is tested—focus, movement, and foot controls. You help coordinate neuro monitoring equipment, preparing needle electrodes (gl) that will track nerve function throughout the procedure.

06:55 — In pre-op, you meet the patient, whose posture reflects years of persistent pain. You introduce yourself and explain your role maintaining the sterile field and supporting the surgeon during the procedure. Their relief is cautious but visible; surgery may not be perfect, but it offers hope.

07:20 — After scrubbing, the patient is positioned prone. Padding, alignment, and verification steps take time—small positioning errors can create serious complications. The timeout confirms identity and procedure, and the incision begins.

07:45 — You pass instruments steadily as the surgeon exposes the lamina (gl) and decompresses nerve roots using Kerrison rongeurs (gl). For the fusion, pedicle screws (gl) and rods are opened and passed. Throughout the procedure, the neuro monitoring technologist calls out updates: "Signals stable," a phrase that quietly reduces tension across the room.

10:30 — Closure begins. Tissue layers are sutured, drains placed, and the patient is transferred carefully to recovery. The room turns over quickly as the next case approaches.

11:10 — The second case—a craniotomy—requires an entirely different setup. Microsurgical instruments, micro scissors, bipolar cautery (gl), and delicate retractors replace the heavier spine trays. The Mayfield clamp (gl) is prepared to stabilize the patient's head.

12:05 — After scrubbing again, neuronavigation (gl) equipment is positioned. When the bone flap (gl) is removed and the dura (gl) appears under the microscope, the room grows quieter. You pass microinstruments and adjust positioning as the surgeon works toward the tumor.

14:20 — Tumor tissue is removed and sent to pathology (gl). The dura is closed, the bone flap secured, and final counts confirmed—sponges, needles, instruments, patties (gl). The patient leaves for ICU monitoring, and the team resets for the final case.

16:00 — A shorter decompression case closes out the day. Even routine procedures require the same vigilance—counts verified, closure completed, and turnover finished.

18:40 — Driving home, the day replays in fragments: the narrow spinal canal (gl) opening during decompression, the stillness of the microscope view, the quiet reassurance when monitoring signals remained steady. Neuro days carry a particular intensity, one that does not fully fade the moment you leave the hospital.

21:20 — Back home, Dash greets you at the door, tail tapping rhythmically against the wall like a metronome finally slowing down. Dinner is simple, conversation minimal, and the body gradually shifts out of procedural focus. Neuro OR days test alignment in a specific way: if working in tiny spaces with enormous stakes energizes you, this environment can feel deeply meaningful. If the weight of that responsibility follows you long after the lights go off, another surgical specialty may ultimately fit better.

Chapter 28

Day In The Life — Rural Hospital

Day in the Life Rural Hospital

05:40 – Your alarm goes off to the sound of birds more than traffic. Working at a rural hospital (gl) means your commute is mostly open road and fields instead of highways and garages. You roll out of bed, stretch your back, and head to the kitchen. Breakfast is simple—something quick but filling. As you eat, you think about today's board the way you always do: a little bit of everything. A gallbladder case, a broken wrist, a C-section "if needed," a possible appendectomy (gl), and one slot that simply reads "open for emergencies."

06:15 – The drive to the hospital is quiet. You badge in, change into scrubs, and store your clothes in a narrow locker along a hallway that feels more clinic-sized than metropolitan hospital-scale.

06:35 – The OR suite here is small—two main rooms and a procedure room off a single hallway. The whiteboard is less crowded than in large centers, but the margin notes tell the real story: "If OB needs us," "Possible ER add-on," "Ortho consult pending." Your assignment reads "OR 1 – General/Ortho," meaning you'll likely move between specialties throughout the day.

Inside OR 1, you prepare the laparoscopic setup for the first case, checking equipment carefully. In smaller facilities, backup trays are limited, so preparation carries extra importance.

07:00 — In pre-op, you meet your first patient—someone you may have seen around town. You introduce yourself and explain your role assisting the surgical team and maintaining the sterile field.

07:25 — The gallbladder case proceeds smoothly. You pass instruments steadily while anesthesia—today a single CRNA covering multiple rooms—monitors the patient. Closure is completed, counts are correct, and the patient moves to recovery.

09:10 — The next case is an open reduction and internal fixation (ORIF) (gl) of a fractured wrist. You open orthopedic trays, preparing plates, screws, and drills. With no dedicated orthopedic tech on shift, you adapt quickly, assisting as needed.

11:30 — Lunch is brief. Conversations in the small break room often include discussions about transfers to larger hospitals when patients require advanced specialty care—another reality of rural practice.

12:05 — The ER calls: suspected appendicitis, possible perforation (gl). Your afternoon schedule shifts immediately.

12:30 — Labor and delivery also alerts the OR that a patient may require a C-section. You prepare a second room while continuing to manage your assigned cases, moving between responsibilities as needed.

14:25 — During the appendectomy, the surgeon converts from laparoscopic to open surgery after finding the appendix perforated. You open additional trays and adjust the setup quickly, passing instruments as the team manages infection and completes the removal.

16:10 — Labor and delivery confirms the C-section. You scrub into the second OR, assisting with the delivery before returning to help reset rooms once the case is complete.

18:00 — The board finally quiets. You restock supplies, prepare instruments for the next day, and receive a quick thank-you from the nurse manager—recognition that in smaller teams, every role carries significant weight.

18:30 — Driving home, you think about the range of cases handled in a single shift: general surgery, orthopedics, emergency procedures, and obstetrics. Rural OR work demands flexibility and independence in ways large facilities rarely do.

21:40 — In bed, you reflect on what rural practice requires: adaptability, teamwork, and the confidence to manage whatever comes through the door. For some clinicians, that unpredictability is exhausting; for others, it is exactly what makes the work meaningful.

SCRUB*fits*™ Reflection — Sergi Tekno

"Turnovers reveal a lot about fit. Some people experience them as chaotic pressure; others experience them as an organizing challenge with a clear objective. If resetting a room quickly and correctly feels energizing rather than draining, that matters."

Chapter 29

Day In The Life — Robotics in the OR

Day in the Life Robotics OR

05:25 — Your alarm goes off and for a second you forget where you are in the rotation. Then you remember: today you are assigned to the robotics (gl) room. Instead of long open incisions, many procedures will be performed through tiny ports while the surgeon operates from a console nearby. You move through your morning routine—shower, breakfast, coffee—with an extra layer of mental checklist running in the background: robot docked and charged, correct instruments pulled, vision cart working, and extra trocars ready. Robotics days are part surgery, part choreography, part technical precision.

06:05 — The hospital parking lot is still half-empty as you pull in. On the board, your name is written next to the robotic room with three cases scheduled: a robotic prostatectomy (gl), a hysterectomy (gl), and a hernia repair. Different specialties—urology (gl) and gynecology (gl)—but the same robotic system waiting in the corner.

06:20 — Inside the room, you uncover the robot, power on the system, and run through the equipment checklist: camera, robotic instruments, insufflator (gl), suction, and electrocautery connections. Robotics setups demand careful preparation because troubleshooting mid-case can delay the entire surgical flow.

06:45 — In pre-op, you meet the first patient and explain that the surgeon will operate using robotic controls while the bedside team remains present to manage instruments and patient safety throughout the procedure.

07:10 — After scrubbing, the patient is positioned in steep Trendelenburg (gl), with careful padding to protect pressure points. You assist with insertion of the Veress needle (gl) or optical trocar (gl), preparing for placement of robotic ports.

07:45 — Once the abdomen is insufflated with CO_2 gas (gl), the robot is rolled into place and docked. Instruments are attached one by one and confirmed on the console display before the surgeon begins operating.

08:15 — The procedure settles into a steady rhythm. You exchange robotic instruments, manage bedside suction, and monitor patient positioning. When the operation is complete, the robot is undocked and closure begins before the patient is transported to recovery.

10:45 — Turnover in a robotics room follows a specific sequence: instruments are sent to sterile processing, robotic tools replaced, and system checks repeated before the next case. You review the next preference card carefully in preparation for the hysterectomy case.

12:05 — The docking sequence repeats for the next procedure, followed later by a smaller robotic hernia repair that completes the day's schedule.

17:40 — After final turnover, you power down the robotic system, cover the arms, document instrument usage, and prepare the room for the next team.

18:45 — Driving home, you reflect on how robotics blends technology with hands-on surgical care. The machines assist the procedure, but setup, troubleshooting, safety checks, and patient reassurance still depend entirely on the human team.

Chapter 30

Day In The Life — Floater

Here is the **glossary-balanced version**, tagging only specialty learning terms at first occurrence and removing unnecessary operational tags.

Day in the Life Float Tech

06:20 — Your alarm goes off with a tone you deliberately chose because it is less jarring. Today you are the float tech (gl), which means you belong to no single room and every room at once. You stretch in bed for an extra few seconds, knowing your day will likely be divided into short bursts of intensity rather than one long case. Breakfast is steady and practical—something that will hold you through multiple room changes. As you eat, you picture the OR board: your name will not be tied to a single surgeon, but to the small note that simply reads "Float."

05:55 — The parking lot is just starting to fill when you arrive. In the core, the whiteboard confirms what you expected: no room assignment, just arrows and shifting responsibilities. The charge nurse gives you the rundown: first breaks in a few rooms, turnovers in others, and likely assistance starting a laparoscopic (gl) case mid-morning.

06:20 — You begin in a general surgery room preparing for a colon resection (gl). The assigned tech is already building the back table, and you help pull additional sutures and supplies before moving to assist another room opening orthopedic trays.

06:50 — Break coverage begins early. In one room, a laparoscopic cholecystectomy (gl) is underway when you step in. After a quick handoff, you pass instruments steadily, anticipating when the clip applier (gl) or retrieval bag will be needed.

07:40 — Another room requires break coverage for a gynecology (gl) procedure, where instruments such as uterine manipulators (gl) and tenaculums (gl) are in use. Float work means shifting quickly between specialties, each with its own rhythm and terminology.

08:25 — You move into turnover support, helping rooms reset quickly for the next cases before heading to assist with a vascular (gl) access procedure for a new dialysis (gl) patient. During the surgery, the team creates a fistula (gl) to support long-term dialysis treatment.

10:45 — Later, you relieve a tech in spine surgery, quickly adjusting to drills, retractors, and implant systems before rotating again to another assignment.

12:40 — The afternoon becomes a sequence of short missions—joint replacement setup, plastics case coverage, and additional turnovers—each requiring quick orientation and immediate readiness.

16:20 — Near the end of the day, you assist briefly in a urology (gl) case before moving on to start another room. The constant transitions are part of the role: flexibility is the skill that matters most.

18:10 — Changing back into your own clothes, you feel a different kind of fatigue than after a long single case—the quieter exhaustion that comes from managing many rooms, many teams, and many shifting responsibilities.

21:10 — In bed, you think again about alignment. Some clinicians prefer the predictability of one room and one specialty. Others find satisfaction in being the person who keeps the entire department moving, stepping in wherever the need is greatest.

SCRUB*fits*™ Reflection — Sergi Tekno

"Surgical technology often rewards quiet excellence. You may not be the person speaking the most in the room, but your work is felt in the smoothness of the case. If being essential without being the center of attention appeals to you, that is a strong alignment marker."

Chapter 31

Day In The Life — Complex Trays and Sterile Processing

Day in the Life Instrument Specialist

05:25 — Your alarm goes off, and for once you do not picture an OR table or a surgical drape as you wake up. Today you are assigned as the instrument specialist, which means most of your work will center around sterile processing (gl) and the most complex surgical trays in the hospital. You still eat a solid breakfast—eggs, toast, coffee—because even though you may not be scrubbed into long cases, this kind of day burns a different kind of energy: walking, lifting, troubleshooting, and constantly solving small puzzles so tomorrow's surgeries are safe and ready.

06:00 — The hospital feels different when you walk past the OR hallway and continue to the lower level, where sterile processing departments are usually located. On the bulletin board, a schedule lists which instrument sets need priority: cardiac (gl) trays, neuro (gl) microsurgical sets, orthopedic (gl) loaner trays (gl) from vendors, and a growing list of items marked "missing" or "needs repair."

06:20 — You begin in the decontamination (gl) area, where used instruments arrive in closed carts. Staff wear full protective equipment while sorting trays and preparing them for washer-disinfectors. You review priority carts, noting any missing clamps, bent forceps, or mismatched loaner components.

06:45 — On the clean side, instruments emerge ready for inspection. You examine a complex laparoscopic (gl) set, checking hinge joints, insulation (gl) on electrosurgical tools, and small attachment pieces that are easy to overlook but essential to safe surgical function.

07:30 — A call comes from the OR about a missing rongeur (gl) in a spine tray. You locate the instrument in a neighboring container and log the correction—preventing a potential delay in the next day's case.

08:15 — You assist newer staff in assembling delicate microvascular (gl) instruments, demonstrating proper protection methods and emphasizing the guiding principle: if you would not want the instrument on your own surgical table, do not send it upstairs.

09:00 — Between cases, OR teams report equipment concerns: a missing ENT (gl) suction component, a malfunctioning sternal saw (gl). You tag items for repair and document them in the tracking system.

10:20 — Back in sterile processing, you update the instrument tracking system (gl) and load autoclaves (gl), placing chemical indicators (gl) appropriately inside each package. After sterilization, integrator strips (gl) are checked to confirm that proper conditions were reached.

12:10 — You conduct an in-service (gl) session with OR staff on new laparoscopic energy devices (gl), demonstrating cleaning procedures and identifying fragile components that require special handling.

13:00 — A shipment of orthopedic loaner trays (gl) arrives for upcoming cases. You verify contents against inventory lists and send the sets through full reprocessing before clinical use.

15:10 — The afternoon becomes a steady rhythm of inspection, assembly, and tray optimization—organizing neuro microsurgical sets, updating cardiac tray layouts, and improving storage access for vascular instruments.

16:30 — End-of-day checks begin. You confirm which trays must be ready for tomorrow's early cases and coordinate priorities with the evening team.

21:00 — In bed, you reflect on how this role produces invisible victories. When trays open perfectly and surgeries start on time, few people think about the preparation behind the scenes—and that quiet reliability is exactly the goal.

Chapter 32

Day In The Life — Traveler Tech

Traveler Tech - First Day at a New Facility

Before the alarm, your **Maine Coon cat Juniper** stretches across the unfamiliar apartment windowsill, watching early headlights move across the street. Traveler housing still feels temporary—neutral walls, rental furniture, and half-unpacked boxes—but Juniper has already claimed the space as home. You scratch behind her ears, reminding yourself that even when everything else changes, small routines travel with you.

05:10 — Your alarm goes off in a bedroom that is not really yours. The walls are bare, the furniture is mismatched, and the kitchen is stocked with exactly the kind of almost-food you buy when you know you will not be here long. This is traveler (gl) housing: functional, temporary, and just personal enough to feel strange when you leave. You lie there for a moment, listening to unfamiliar pipes and distant traffic, and remind yourself that this is what you signed up for—new city, new hospital, new OR. You swing your legs over the side of the bed and head for the kitchen.

05:30 — Breakfast is quiet. There is no roommate or partner walking through, no familiar routine yet. Just you, a mug of coffee, and something simple you can eat quickly—toast, eggs, maybe yogurt. On your phone, you open the email from your agency with your assignment details: facility name, unit, arrival time, contact person. "Report to OR front desk at 06:30," it says. "Ask for charge nurse." You recheck the address even though you memorized it last night. First days are not the time to improvise.

06:05 — The drive to the hospital introduces you to your new city in snapshots: small restaurants, a park you might visit once, a skyline that still feels temporary. The hospital rises ahead of you, larger than expected. Inside, you check in at security, receive a temporary badge, and wait while a clerk prints your permanent ID with your name and "Travel ST" under it.

06:25 — At the OR front desk, everything feels both familiar and unfamiliar. You introduce yourself to the charge nurse, who assigns you to OR 7 with general surgery. "You'll have a short orientation and then work with a preceptor (gl) for the first cases," she says. Relief settles in—you will not be completely on your own yet.

06:40 — In the locker room, you change into hospital-issued scrubs, noticing the color is different from your last assignment. A staff tech introduces herself and walks you through the core, pointing out supply rooms, case cart flow, and how this facility organizes preference cards (gl). Small differences matter; learning them quickly is part of traveler life.

07:05 — OR 7 prepares for a laparoscopic (gl) cholecystectomy (gl). The setup feels familiar, but supply locations are different. The staff tech narrates the surgeon's preferences—specific trocars (gl), camera cords, and table layout. You map the room mentally while assisting with setup.

07:30 — In pre-op, you meet the first patient and introduce yourself as part of the surgical team. Their anxiety looks the same as patients everywhere; your calm tone matters more than where you are from.

07:50 — Back in the OR, you scrub in. Your preceptor runs the first case while you observe the surgeon's rhythm and local workflow. By the second case, you begin taking the lead, pulling supplies, opening instruments, and rebuilding your muscle memory within a new environment.

11:45 — Lunch introduces you to the OR culture. Staff ask where your last contracts were, and the conversation shifts from cautious curiosity to casual inclusion.

12:20 — The afternoon brings an unexpected assignment: assisting with a knee arthroscopy (gl). The trays differ slightly from those at previous hospitals, but the fundamentals remain the same—watch the monitor, anticipate instruments, keep the field organized.

15:10 — A small hernia repair closes the scheduled day. This time, the supplies feel easier to find, and your setup flows more naturally. Each case makes the environment less unfamiliar.

16:30 — Before leaving, the charge nurse walks you through emergency tray locations, after-hours workflows, and sterile processing (gl) contact procedures—practical knowledge that determines whether tomorrow runs smoothly.

17:15 — In the locker room, you change back into your own clothes. You still feel like the new person, but less than you did this morning.

18:30 — At the apartment, Juniper greets you at the door as if nothing changed. You eat dinner, answer a few "How was day one?" texts, and think about the trade traveler life requires: flexibility, constant adaptation, and proving yourself repeatedly.

21:40 — In bed, you mentally walk through the hospital layout one more time—entrance, OR desk, supply rooms, OR 7. First days rarely feel smooth, but they reveal something important: whether you can see yourself lasting day ten, day fifty, day ninety. Tonight, your answer is a steady, cautious: "I can work with this."

SCRUB*fits*™ Reflection — Sergi Tekno

"The OR runs on precision under time constraints. If you find satisfaction in details — counts, field organization, instrument readiness, and anticipating needs — you may thrive in roles where accuracy is the foundation of speed."

Chapter 33
Salary and Job Market Guide

There are two conversations happening in the operating room at all times. One is clinical — instruments, anatomy, sequence. The other is invisible — staffing, shortages, compensation, and the economic reality of running a surgical service. Most students only hear the first. This chapter gives you both. It is not enough to know how to scrub in. You deserve to know where this career can take you financially, what hospitals are willing to pay for your skill set, and why certain regions and specialties are at a constant simmer of "we need more people — now." This is your full guide to the salary landscape of Surgical Technology: where you can earn the most, where the shortages are deepest, and how to think about money in a way that actually supports alignment rather than draining it.

The Big Picture: What Surgical Technologists Earn Nationwide

Across the country, Surgical Technologists sit in a remarkably stable pay range — stronger than many other allied health roles with similar training requirements. National data show the median annual wage clustered around the mid-$50,000s to mid-$60,000s, depending on region, specialty, and experience. But here's the part that matters: the range is wide — from the low $40,000s in underfunded regions to the high $80,000s or even $90,000s in specialty-heavy markets. Your location and specialty matter more than your graduation date. Much more.

Where Surgical Technologists Earn the Most

Certain states unlock dramatically higher wages for Surgical Technologists — and it's not random. It's where demand outruns supply, operating room volume is high, complex specialties dominate, hospitals pay more to stay afloat, and cost-of-living (gl) increases pressure to recruit. The following regions consistently land at or near the top:

1 **Alaska** — Frontier healthcare, limited workforce, and high-demand OR environments push pay into the high $70,000s to low $80,000s.

2 **California** — High cost-of-living, union presence in some systems, and major surgical volume mean experienced STs regularly hit $80,000–$90,000, with even higher earning potential in certain specialties or call-heavy services.

3 **Washington & Oregon** — Strong hospital networks and expanding surgical centers place STs in the mid-$60,000s to high $70,000s, with specialty rooms pushing beyond that.

4 **Nevada, Colorado, Massachusetts, New York** — Diverse surgical ecosystems and competition among health systems drive pay into the upper $60,000s and beyond.

But salary alone is not the story. Once you factor in price of housing, groceries, taxes, and transportation, some "average pay" states outrank the "big pay" ones in real quality of life.

The Real Question: What Does Your Salary Buy You Here?

A Surgical Technologist making $57,000 in a lower-cost state may live a more stable, less stressful life than a Surgical Technologist making $82,000 in a high-cost metro area. Your alignment (gl) depends not on how big the number looks, but how hard you must grind to survive. A $2,000 rent payment can turn a good job into a trap. A $900 rent payment can turn the same salary into breathing room. This is why we always evaluate salary, cost-of-living, commute, housing stability, call expectations, shift structure, burnout risk, and lifestyle impact. Money is only helpful if it supports your life — not if it devours it.

How Specialty Affects Your Pay

Not all surgeries pay the same. Not all surgeons want the same skill set. And the more specialized the room, the more hospitals will pay to get someone who can walk in and scrub without hesitation. High-paying specialties include cardiothoracic surgery, neurosurgery, orthopedics, trauma, robotics, plastics, ENT, and spine. If you want to maximize your income in this field, specialty matters more than tenure.

What About Travel Surgical Technologists?

Travel Surgical Technologists are the wild card in the salary landscape. Travelers often earn $1,500–$2,500 per week, or roughly $65,000–$110,000+ per year equivalent, depending on the market, acuity, and stipends. Some markets spike even higher during shortages or peak seasons. Travel STs can significantly accelerate loan payoff, savings goals, down payments, and career exploration. But the trade-offs are real: constant onboarding, no long-term team relationships, variable housing, unpredictable contract changes, and high pressure to adapt instantly. Travel can be perfect for a season of your life — just not usually a lifetime.

Where the Shortages Are — And Why They Matter

Shortages are not equal across the country. Some regions are overwhelmed with OR openings because the population is aging, surgical volume is rising, hospitals expanded faster than their workforce, retirement rates outpace graduation rates, burnout is pushing people out, and new surgical centers are opening faster than they can staff. The deepest shortages for Surgical Technologists tend to be in rural hospitals in the Midwest and South, underserved regions, large urban trauma centers, fast-growing Sunbelt cities, and surgical centers competing with hospitals for talent. Shortage equals leverage — and opportunity — including faster hiring, higher starting pay, relocation packages, tuition support, faster advancement, and higher specialty exposure. But remember: shortage pay often signals high strain. Don't chase money into misalignment.

Shift Differentials: The Secret Income Boost

Shift structure is a hidden pay multiplier. You can significantly increase your income by working evenings, choosing weekend shifts, taking consistent call, joining trauma or ortho rotation teams, working holidays strategically, or picking units with high overtime availability. Some STs boost their income by 20–30% purely through strategic shift choices. But again, the trade-off belongs in your alignment equation.

What New Graduates Earn vs. What Experienced STs Earn

New graduates typically start in the low-to-mid $40,000s to low $50,000s depending on location and specialty. Mid-career STs often move into the mid-$50,000s to low $70,000s with experience and certification. Specialty-focused STs in cardiothoracic, neuro, or robotics regularly reach $70,000–$90,000 in high-demand markets. Travel STs may exceed $100,000 with stipends and overtime. Experience multiplies income far more than tenure.

Bonuses, Incentives, and Additional Pay

Hospitals may offer sign-on bonuses, retention bonuses, relocation assistance, tuition reimbursement, call pay, certification pay, specialty premiums, and internal float pool rates. The more flexible you are, the higher your ceiling.

Alignment + Money: Your Best Decision-Making Filter

Pay is one part of the career. Meaning is another. Protection is another. Alignment is the most powerful filter you have. Ask yourself: "Where can I earn enough and still live a life that feels like mine?" If a job pays more but costs you your health, sleep, sanity, or relationships, it is not a good trade. If a job pays a little less but gives you predictability, a supportive team, a specialty you love, and a sustainable schedule, that is often worth far more over time.

The Long View: What Real Wealth Looks Like for STs

Wealth for a Surgical Technologist is less about chasing massive pay spikes and more about choosing specialty intentionally, managing burnout risk, stacking certifications, using relocation or shift differentials strategically, avoiding lifestyle creep, protecting your physical health, and choosing teams that help you stay in the field longer. Some STs earn more in five years than others earn in fifteen — not because they are better, but because they made aligned choices early.

The Bottom Line

Surgical Technology can be financially stable, upwardly mobile, specialty flexible, geographically flexible, and full of opportunities. The key is to know the landscape before you enter it. When you understand the interplay of specialty, geography, shift structure, and shortages, you stop thinking, "What will they offer me?" and start thinking, "Where do my skills, my wiring, and my life come together best?" That moment — the moment you negotiate from alignment — is the moment you stop surviving your career and start shaping it.

Chapter 34
The Never End

Every healthcare career has a beginning, but the meaningful ones never really have a final chapter. They evolve, expand, and reshape themselves as you grow — through new skills, new specialties, new teams, and new versions of who you become along the way. Surgical Technology is no different. What begins as learning to maintain a sterile field and pass instruments with precision can eventually become leadership in the operating room, advanced specialty expertise, teaching future techs, traveling across the country, or stepping into entirely new healthcare pathways built on the foundation you have created.

If this guide has done its job, you now understand far more than what a Surgical Technologist does. You understand the rhythm of the operating room, the physical and emotional demands of the role, the financial landscape, the hiring process, the specialties that shape long-term careers, and the alignment questions that matter most before committing to this path. Most importantly, you understand that choosing a healthcare career is not simply about what you *can* do, but about where your personality, stamina, priorities, and long-term goals fit best.

Throughout this book, you met the **SCRUB*fits*™**—not as mascots, but as reminders that people thrive in different environments for different reasons. Some professionals feel most alive in fast trauma rooms. Others find purpose in steady outpatient procedures, robotics programs, cardiac teams, or rural hospitals where versatility defines the role. There is no single "right" version of Surgical Technology. There is only the version that aligns with who you are and the life you want to build.

As you move forward, remember that your first job is not your final destination. Early roles are classrooms. Each service line you learn, each surgeon you work with, each specialty you experience becomes part of your professional vocabulary. Over time, those experiences give you options — and options create freedom. The goal is not just to enter the field, but to build a career that you can sustain, grow within, and remain proud of many years from now.

If you ever find yourself questioning whether you still belong in a particular room, specialty, or environment, return to the same alignment questions you asked at the beginning:

Where do I work best?

What pace strengthens me instead of draining me?

What teams help me grow?

What kind of day leaves me tired in a good way?

Those questions will continue guiding you long after your first credential, your first job, or even your first promotion. Careers evolve, and so will you.

Thank you for spending this time with me, for exploring the world of Surgical Technology with honesty and curiosity, and for taking your future seriously enough to ask not only *"Can I do this?"* but also *"Is this where I belong?"* Wherever your path leads next — the OR, another specialty, advanced training, or a new direction entirely — remember that alignment is not a one-time decision. It is a lifelong conversation between who you are and the work you choose to do.

This is not the end of the story. It is simply the page where your next chapter begins.

Goodbye for now.

StaySm:)in'!

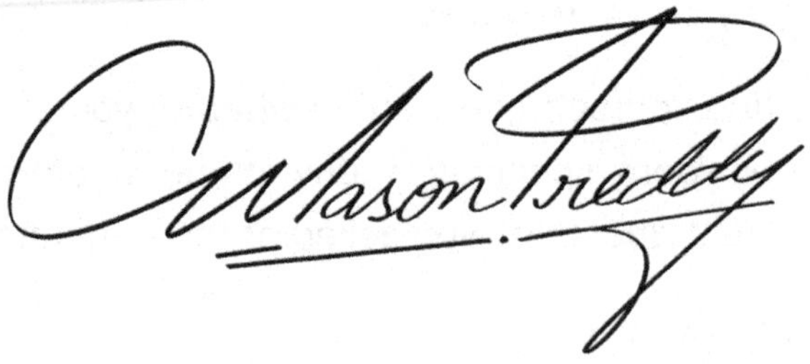

Chapter 35

Surgical Technologist Glossary

(gl)

1. Aseptic Technique

Practices used to prevent contamination by microorganisms during surgical procedures. (Infection Prevention / OR Practice / Core)

2. Autoclave

A pressurized steam sterilizer used to eliminate microorganisms on surgical instruments and supplies. (Sterile Processing / Equipment / Core)

3. Back Table

The sterile workspace where surgical instruments and supplies are organized during a procedure. (OR Workflow / Equipment / Core)

4. Biopsy

Removal of tissue for diagnostic examination. (Surgical Procedure / Diagnostic / Core)

5. Case Cart

A transport cart containing all supplies and instruments prepared for a specific surgical procedure. (OR Workflow / Logistics / Core)

6. Circulating Nurse

A non-sterile team member responsible for patient advocacy, documentation, and obtaining additional supplies during surgery. (OR Roles / Teamwork / Core)

7. Count

The process of verifying that all surgical instruments, sponges, and sharps are accounted for before, during, and after a procedure. (Safety / OR Protocol / Core)

8. Draping

Placement of sterile coverings around the surgical site to maintain a sterile field. (OR Procedure / Sterility / Core)

9. Electrocautery

A device that uses electrical current to cut tissue or control bleeding. (Surgical Equipment / Energy Devices / Core)

10. Endoscope

A camera-equipped instrument inserted into the body to visualize internal structures. (Minimally Invasive Surgery / Equipment / Core)

11. Forceps

Handheld instruments used for grasping, holding, or manipulating tissue. (Surgical Instruments / Core)

12. Hemostasis

Control of bleeding during surgery. (Surgical Principles / Clinical / Core)

13. Implant

A medical device or material placed inside the body during surgery. (Surgical Materials / Specialty / Core)

14. Instrument Tray

A standardized set of surgical instruments assembled for a specific procedure. (Sterile Processing / Equipment / Core)

15. Laparoscopic Surgery

Minimally invasive surgery performed using small incisions and camera-guided instruments. (Surgical Technique / Core)

16. Mayo Stand

A movable sterile stand positioned over the patient to hold frequently used instruments. (OR Equipment / Workflow / Core)

17. Mesh

Synthetic or biologic material used to reinforce tissue, commonly in hernia repairs. (Surgical Materials / General Surgery / Core)

18. Preference Card

A documented list of a surgeon's preferred instruments,

supplies, and setup for procedures. (OR Workflow / Documentation / Core)

19. Retractor

An instrument used to hold back tissue or organs to improve surgical visibility. (Surgical Instruments / Core)

20. Scrub In

The surgical hand antisepsis process performed before donning sterile gown and gloves. (Sterility / OR Protocol / Core)

21. Sterile Field

The designated sterile area that includes instruments, supplies, and the surgical site. (Infection Prevention / OR Practice / Core)

22. Sterile Processing

The department responsible for cleaning, assembling, sterilizing, and distributing surgical instruments. (Hospital Operations / Core)

23. Suction

Equipment used to remove fluids such as blood from the surgical field. (Surgical Equipment / Core)

24. Suture

Material used to close wounds or surgical incisions. (Surgical Materials / Core)

25. Trocar

A sharp instrument inserted through the abdominal wall to allow entry of laparoscopic instruments. (Minimally Invasive Surgery / Equipment / Core)

26. Turnover

The process of cleaning, restocking, and preparing an operating room between cases. (OR Workflow / Operations / Core)

27. Vendor Tray

A loaned instrument set provided by medical device companies for specialized procedures. (Supply Chain / OR Logistics / Core)

28. Wound Closure

The final surgical step involving sutures, staples, or adhesives to close tissue layers. (Surgical Technique / Core)

29. Surgical Time-Out

A safety pause conducted before incision to confirm patient identity, procedure, and surgical site. (Patient Safety / Protocol / Core)

30. Surgical Count Sheet

Documentation used to track instrument, sponge, and sharp counts during procedures. (Safety / Documentation / Core)

31. Instrument Stringer

A device used to hold ring-handled instruments open during sterilization. (Sterile Processing / Equipment / Core)

32. Biological Indicator

A testing device used to confirm that sterilization processes effectively destroyed microorganisms. (Sterility Assurance / Quality Control / Core)

33. Sterile Packaging

Materials used to wrap or containerize instruments to maintain sterility until use. (Sterile Processing / Logistics / Core)

34. Positioning

Placement of the patient on the operating table to optimize surgical access and prevent injury. (Patient Safety / OR Practice / Core)

35. Surgical Sponge

Absorbent material used to control bleeding and maintain visibility in the surgical field. (Surgical Supplies / Core)

36. Robotic Surgery System

Computer-assisted surgical equipment allowing surgeons to operate using robotic-controlled instruments. (Advanced Technology / Specialty / Core)

37. Contaminated

A state in which sterile items or fields are exposed to microorganisms and are no longer considered sterile. (Infection Prevention / Core)

38. Flash Sterilization

Rapid sterilization process used for urgent reprocessing of instruments. (Sterile Processing / Operations / Core)

39. Surgical Consent

Formal patient authorization for a surgical procedure after explanation of risks and benefits. (Legal / Patient Rights / Core)

40. Surgical Specimen

Tissue or material removed during surgery and sent for laboratory analysis. (Pathology / Surgical Workflow / Core)

Bonus Glossary — Surgical Technologist

Introduction

Surgical technology is a precision-driven profession built on specialized terminology that reflects the rhythm, safety standards, and teamwork of the operating room. Becoming fluent in this language is not simply academic; it allows surgical technologists to anticipate surgeon needs, communicate clearly with the perioperative team, and maintain the sterile environment that protects patients. The following bonus glossary introduces 100 additional foundational terms that every aspiring or practicing Surgical Technologist should begin learning early. Mastery of these concepts strengthens situational awareness, improves workflow efficiency, and supports the high-reliability performance expected inside modern operating suites.

100 Essential Bonus Terms

1 Aseptic Technique — Methods used to prevent contamination by microorganisms.

2 Back Table — Sterile table where instruments and supplies are organized for the procedure.

3 **Bioburden** — Microorganisms present on instruments prior to sterilization.

4 **Case Cart** — Cart containing supplies needed for a scheduled surgical procedure.

5 **Circulator** — Non-sterile nurse who manages room coordination and documentation.

6 **Clamp** — Instrument used to occlude vessels or grasp tissue.

7 **Count Sheet** — Document used to track surgical instruments and sponges.

8 **Debridement** — Removal of damaged or dead tissue.

9 **Draping** — Placement of sterile coverings to isolate the operative field.

10 **Electrocautery** — Device using electric current to cut tissue or control bleeding.

11 **Endoscope** — Instrument used to visualize internal structures through small incisions.

12 **Field Contamination** — Breach in sterile conditions.

13 **Forceps** — Instrument used for grasping or holding tissue.

14 **Gowning** — Donning sterile surgical attire.

15 **Hemostasis** — Control of bleeding.

16 **Implant Log** — Record documenting implanted medical devices.

17 **Instrument Stringer** — Rack used for organizing ring-handled instruments during sterilization.

18 Laparoscope — Endoscopic device used in minimally invasive surgery.

19 Mayo Stand — Adjustable sterile stand holding frequently used instruments.

20 Needle Driver — Instrument used to hold suturing needles.

21 Operating Field — Area where the surgical procedure occurs.

22 Peel Pack — Individually wrapped sterile instrument package.

23 Prep Solution — Antiseptic solution used to disinfect skin before surgery.

24 Retractor — Instrument used to hold back tissue for exposure.

25 Sponge Stick — Instrument used to hold sponges during prepping.

26 Sterile Barrier — Protective covering maintaining sterility.

27 Suction Tip — Device used to remove fluids from the surgical field.

28 Surgical Timeout — Final safety verification before incision.

29 Trocar — Instrument used to create entry ports in minimally invasive surgery.

30 Wrapping Technique — Method used to prepare instruments for sterilization.

31 Autoclave — Machine using steam to sterilize instruments.

32 Basin Set — Sterile containers used to hold solutions.

33 Case Pick List — Inventory list of required surgical supplies.

34 Contaminated Item — Object that has lost sterility.

35 Disposable Drapes — Single-use sterile coverings.

36 Exposure — Visibility of the surgical site.

37 Field Setup — Arrangement of sterile instruments before surgery.

38 Glove Integrity — Condition of sterile gloves remaining intact.

39 Hand Hygiene Protocol — Required hand-cleansing procedures.

40 Indicator Tape — Tape confirming sterilization exposure.

41 Kick Bucket — Container for discarded surgical waste.

42 Ligation — Tying off vessels to stop bleeding.

43 Mesh Implant — Synthetic material used for tissue reinforcement.

44 Neutral Zone — Area for safe passing of sharps.

45 Open Gloving — Technique for donning sterile gloves individually.

46 Pack Integrity — Assurance sterile packaging remains intact.

47 Positioning Devices — Equipment used to safely position patients.

48 Procedure Preference Card — Surgeon-specific supply list.

49 Ring Forceps — Instrument used to hold sponges or materials.

50 Scrub Sink — Designated area for surgical hand antisepsis.

51 Sharps Container — Disposal unit for needles and blades.

52 Skin Prep — Antiseptic cleansing of the operative site.

53 Specimen Cup — Container used to collect surgical specimens.

54 Sterility Indicator — Device confirming sterilization success.

55 Surgical Blade — Detachable scalpel blade.

56 Table Height Adjustment — Positioning table for ergonomic workflow.

57 Turnover Time — Time required to prepare the room for the next case.

58 Utility Drape — Drape with adhesive opening for incision area.

59 Vessel Loop — Silicone loop used to control vessels.

60 Wound Closure Kit — Supplies used for closing surgical incisions.

61 Air Exchange Rate — Frequency of air replacement in the OR.

62 Biohazard Waste — Waste contaminated with infectious materials.

63 Chemical Indicator Strip — Strip verifying sterilization conditions.

64 Disposable Suction Tubing — Single-use tubing for fluid removal.

65 End-of-Case Count — Final instrument and sponge verification.

66 Fluid Management System — Equipment controlling surgical irrigation fluids.

67 Gauze Count — Accounting of all surgical gauze used.

68 Hand-Off Communication — Transfer of patient care information.

69 Implant Verification — Confirmation of correct implant type and size.

70 Instrument Tray — Organized container of surgical tools.

71 Joint Commission Standards — National healthcare safety regulations.

72 Laser Safety Protocol — Procedures for safe surgical laser use.

73 Medication Labeling — Proper identification of sterile medications.

74 Negative Pressure Room — Room designed to prevent airborne spread.

75 OR Core — Central sterile supply area adjacent to operating rooms.

76 Patient Identification Band — Wristband confirming patient identity.

77 Quality Assurance Audit — Review of compliance with standards.

78 Recovery Transfer Sheet — Document used when transferring patients post-procedure.

79 Safety Checklist — Pre-procedure verification document.

80 Specimen Labeling Protocol — Correct identification of collected specimens.

81 Sterile Field Monitoring — Continuous observation for contamination risks.

82 Surgical Light Handle Cover — Sterile cover for overhead light adjustment.

83 Tissue Forceps — Forceps designed for delicate tissue handling.

84 Transport Gurney — Mobile stretcher used for patient movement.

85 Universal Precautions — Infection-control measures applied to all patients.

86 Vacuum Sealed Pack — Sterile packaging method.

87 Warming Blanket System — Device used to maintain patient body temperature.

88 X-Ray Detectable Sponge — Sponge containing radiopaque marker.

89 Yield Testing — Evaluation of sterilization effectiveness.

90 Zone Cleaning Protocol — Structured OR environmental cleaning process.

91 Allis Clamp — Grasping instrument used on tough tissue.

92 Bulldog Clamp — Small vascular clamp for temporary occlusion.

93 Curette — Instrument used for scraping tissue.

94 Dilator — Instrument used to enlarge an opening.

95 Eschar — Dead tissue resulting from burns.

96 Fascia — Connective tissue layer covering muscles.

97 Hemostat — Instrument used to clamp blood vessels.

98 Irrigation Syringe — Device used to flush wounds or cavities.

99 Jackson-Pratt Drain — Closed suction drainage device.

100 Knot Pusher — Instrument used in minimally invasive suturing.

About the Author

Mason Preddy brings more than 25 years of experience in healthcare recruitment, retention, and workforce strategy to his writing, working closely with hospitals, health systems, academic institutions, and clinical leaders across the United States. Throughout his career, he has helped thousands of healthcare professionals navigate career decisions, specialty transitions, and long-term professional growth, giving him a unique inside view of how clinical roles truly function beyond job descriptions.

He is the creator of Mason's Alignment Theory (MAT) and the developer of the alignment-focused **SCRUB*fit*™** career framework, designed to help healthcare professionals choose roles that match their personality, strengths, lifestyle needs, and long-term sustainability. His work focuses on reducing burnout, improving retention, and helping individuals build healthcare careers that are both professionally rewarding and personally sustainable.

Mason is the founder of Mason Maison™ Publishing and the author of *What Color Are Your Scrubs?* along with the ScrubTales™ career-guide series, which provides real-world, day-in-the-life insight into healthcare professions. His mission is simple: help people **find their fit before they commit**, so that the next generation of healthcare professionals enters the field informed, aligned, and prepared for the realities of modern clinical practice.

Also by Mason Maison™ Publishing

What Color Are Your Scrubs?

A comprehensive career exploration guide covering 345 healthcare careers, designed to help students, career changers, and early-career professionals understand the realities of healthcare roles, identify alignment using structured decision frameworks, and choose pathways that support long-term sustainability and purpose.

ScrubTales™ Series — Real-World Career Guides to Healthcare Professions

A growing collection of cinematic, day-in-the-life career guides that take readers inside healthcare roles through immersive storytelling, practical hiring guidance, financial insights, and alignment-focused decision tools. Each volume explores the lived reality of a specific profession, helping readers understand not only what the job requires, but what it truly feels like to live it.

Visit **MasonMaison.pub** to explore current and upcoming titles, resources, and alignment-focused healthcare career tools.